succeeding

as a

general
practitioner

the experts share
their secrets

Edited by Dr Ian Bogle

HEALTH PRESS

Succeeding as a General Practitioner
First published 2002

© 2002 in this edition Health Press Limited
Health Press Limited, Elizabeth House, Queen Street, Abingdon, Oxford OX14 3JR, UK
Tel: +44 (0)1235 523233
Fax: +44 (0)1235 523238

A CIP catalogue record for this title is available from the British Library.

ISBN 1-903734-09-6

Bogle, I (Ian)
Succeeding as a General Practitioner/
Ian Bogle

Typeset by Zed, Oxford, UK
Printed by Fine Print (Services) Ltd, Oxford, UK

Contents

the editor's introduction

Dr Ian Bogle, Chairman of the Council,
British Medical Association

Like his father before him, my father practised as a GP in inner-city Liverpool for most of his working life. When I ignored his advice, rejected a career in hospital medicine and went into practice alongside him 38 years ago I did so for one simple reason – I wanted to help people who were ill and in distress.

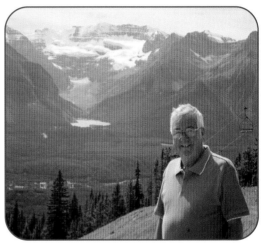

I was brought up in the city. I saw with my own eyes the deprivation and desperation that caused so much misery and suffering and blighted so many lives. I wanted to practise family medicine. I wanted to get to know my patients, and to treat them in their own environment. I wanted to treat people, not diseases. General practice was my vocation.

My grandfather George set up practice in Liverpool in 1911, at a time when childhood morbidity and mortality were high and ailments we now regard as minor and easily treatable could be killers. He was a well-known and respected local figure, revered and deferred to by his patients. In those days, there was no question of a doctor involving a patient in decision-making about their care or treatment. What we now like to call 'consensus medicine' simply didn't exist. Patients neither expected nor demanded anything more than being

> I wanted to **treat people,**
> not **diseases**

told what was wrong with them and being told what their doctor was going to do about it. My grandfather practised in an age when paternalism and instruction were expected and accepted. Patients did as they were told, and his judgement and his choice of treatment were never questioned.

The first Dr Bogle was his own man with all the time in the world to practise medicine. His consultations were long and involved, and he did his home visits on a bicycle. Nevertheless, his weekdays and weekends were full. He was permanently on-call, although at that time patients didn't have phones so very rarely called out their GP at night.

There was of course no National Heath Service, and for many years my grandfather's only member of staff was a debt collector. His social conscience often got the better of him when it came to charging patients, and I am reliably informed that well-off patients were often over-charged and poorer patients were charged very little or nothing. I was once told by a former patient of his that when he was visiting poorer households he would sometimes dip into his pocket and leave money for them if he thought they were having trouble making ends meet. On the surface he was a rather rude and formidable Scotsman, but underneath he was someone who cared a great deal about his patients and would go to great lengths for them.

My grandfather and father were staunch supporters of the introduction of the NHS, if only for the reason that they would no longer have to make financial judgements about their patients and could get on with giving all of them the care they deserved regardless of their economic circumstances.

Nationally, there was a lack of enthusiasm among GPs and hospital doctors for the NHS in the lead-up to its introduction, even though the British Medical Association had put forward its own proposals along similar lines some 3 years before. The level of taxable income declared by GPs prior to the formation of the NHS was used as a baseline for determining payments to GPs contracted to work in the NHS, and it was felt by family doctors at large that these payments were set too low from the outset. Reluctantly, GPs as a body agreed to the new arrangements and were drawn into the NHS while retaining their status as independent contractors. Perhaps it is only now, as more and more work continues to be piled onto primary care and GPs' income falls further and further behind that of comparable professionals, that we have come to realize that as a profession we have always sold ourselves short.

GP pay remained at a very low level until 1950, when galloping post-war inflation and protests to government from the profession prompted the setting up of an independent inquiry, which recommended a substantial pay increase. A royal commission on the NHS followed in the late 1950s, and included among its recommendations the establishment of an independent pay-review body for doctors to set pay levels and make recommendations to government. NHS doctors' pay continues to be determined in this way.

The 1966 GP Charter was the first great watershed in NHS general practice. For doctors of my generation it marked the beginning of a 20-year golden age for general practice in which practising as a family doctor was at its most satisfying and rewarding. The GP Charter revolutionized general practice, heralding the end of one-man bands and the beginning of primary care teams as we know them today. It brought in the ancillary staff reimbursement scheme, the notional rent scheme, and consolidated GP expenses as part of gross income. The revamping of the Red Book and the introduction of the basic practice allowance encouraged doctors to group together to deliver services to patients.

It was not long after this that the College of General Practitioners was granted Chartered status. The College had been formed in 1952 to help raise the standards and status of general practice and encourage medical students to regard general practice as a specialism that could offer an interesting and rewarding career.

When I went into practice there was an assumption among patients that doctors only became GPs if they weren't good enough to do anything else. The coming of the College, and later the introduction of vocational training for general practice, did much to alter the perception of general practice among the public and potential entrants to the specialty.

General practice hit the buffers in the mid-1980s when the Thatcher administration, driven by a desire to gain more control over an independent contractor workforce

General practice hit the buffers in the mid-1980s

and cash limit GP expenditure, set about shaking up GP and community nursing services with the stated aim of placing primary care at the forefront of the health service. Attempts to remove GPs' staff budgets were thwarted by BMA negotiators, but the Conservatives' desire to exercise more control over general practice led ultimately to the imposition of the infamous 1990 GP contract, under which family doctors remained Red Book independent contractors but were saddled with stiflingly bureaucratic administrative responsibilities and required to meet meaningless targets for cervical cytology, immunization and health promotion activity. At a stroke, GPs were expected to take responsibility for the care of a whole community on top of their obligation to individual patients. The profession's representatives spent the early 1990s attempting to remove or renegotiate parts of the contract that were a nonsense.

The introduction of the NHS internal market and GP fundholding cast family doctors once more in the role of businessmen, expected to balance budgets and negotiate on behalf of their patients for services. A BMA survey of all doctors working in general practice at this time identified four priorities for the future.

- New ways of delivering GP out-of-hours services and appropriate payment for out-of-hours work.
- Contractual options other than independent contractor status and the provision of general medical services through the Red Book.
- Identification of core services every NHS GP should be expected to provide in order to halt the uncontrolled shift of work from secondary to primary care, and to ensure GPs received appropriate payment for new work.
- The introduction of a system of reaccreditation for GPs.

All four have either been delivered or are in the process of being delivered. The most significant of these has been the change in the delivery of out-of-hours services as a result of new arrangements negotiated by the BMA in 1995. The agreement precipitated a shift away from a visiting culture to a recognition that patients who need to see a GP urgently, but who are able to travel, are best treated at designated out-of-hours emergency centres that are properly staffed and equipped. The establishment of out-of-hours cooperatives using telephone triage, extra funding enabling GPs to use commercial deputizing services to provide out-of-hours cover and special aid for isolated practitioners have eased the burden on a GP workforce whose workload is increasing inexorably.

The Blair administration has done what the Conservatives threatened to do and cash-limited a demand-led service. Now practices work within budgets through primary care groups and primary care trusts, and the money for patient care is in the same pot as the money for prescribing. The price of pharmaceuticals is not within doctors' control, and when they go over budget, as they often do, something has to give.

In recent years, a more informed and demanding public coupled with the publicity generated by a handful of high-profile misconduct cases have put doctors' competence and accountability under the microscope. Doctors themselves have recognized the need for a more robust and transparent performance review system that commands the confidence of the public and politicians. The General Medical Council, in consultation with the leaders of the profession, is developing a system of revalidation under which continued registration for all doctors will depend on regular demonstration of fitness to practise.

The readiness of ministers and the media to seize on exceptional cases and present them as representative of the profession as a whole has had a dangerously damaging effect on doctors' morale. Today, GPs practising in the NHS, like their colleagues in hospital medicine, are working under greater pressure than ever before. They are working in an environment where they are wary of taking risks, wary of going out on a limb for patients, and wary even to practise good medicine for fear of the backlash if anything goes wrong.

> Today **GPs in the NHS** are **working under greater pressure** than ever before

As for the future, if revalidation is introduced successfully it will relieve some of the pressure the profession is under.

GPs will work under a variety of contractual arrangements, and there will undoubtedly be a shift away from the Red Book as a mechanism for paying GPs and a move towards identifying quality indicators that will be the basis of enhanced pay. There has already been a move away from Kenneth Clarke's obsession with capitation-based payments, and further movement is inevitable.

Patients want and need more time with doctors. Doctors want and need more time with patients. Nowadays, the patient who gets more than 8 minutes with their GP is the lucky one. We must find a way of making more time for patients, and that will mean attracting more young doctors into general practice and persuading older doctors back into general practice. It will mean thinking seriously about skill mix, and about new and enhanced roles for nurses and other members of the primary care team.

More than 90% of doctor–patient contacts in the NHS occur in general practice. In the majority of cases, GPs are the first, and often the only, contact the public has with the health service. The relationship between a patient and their GP is a unique and precious one, built on trust, confidence and mutual respect.

> If the **patient** in front of me **were** my **child, wife, mother** or **father,** what would I want for them?

When making a decision about how to treat someone, I have always asked myself the same question. If the patient in front of me were my child, my wife, my mother or father, what would I want for them?

Society is changing, and what patients expect of us is changing. But one thing hasn't changed, and I'm sure will never change – the instinct of doctors to put their patients first.

skills and attributes of a GP

Dr Colin Tidy, GP

The skills required of the GP have always been diverse, but this is increasingly the case in the current era of rapid change. The intensifying expectations of patients, the culture of evidence-based medicine and the increasing requirements of primary healthcare are all adding to the pressure on general practice. Set against this is the move towards greater teamwork and more appropriate use of the skill mix of not only GPs, but also nurses, counsellors and other allied health professionals.

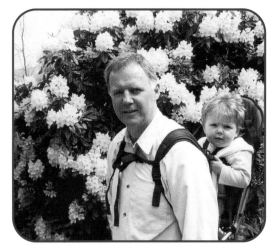

We are also no different from the rest of society in looking for a better balance between career and leisure time with family and friends. The advent of cooperatives and other methods of on-call provision, away from the traditional practice-based rota, have enabled the GP to plan for more complete leisure time than has been the case in the past. More and

> **GPs** are looking for a better **balance** between **career** and **leisure**

more GPs are either working part-time or developing other career interests alongside general practice, and this can also help to reduce the stress and potential 'burn out' that can result from excessive demands. The benefits and strength of general practice have been based largely on its diversity and, although standards of healthcare need to become more consistent, our individual work patterns are becoming ever more varied.

Interacting with the patient

Although we all learn detailed methods of history-taking and examination at medical school, there is never enough time for these to be followed in primary care with, at best, 10 minutes for each patient. The central ability of the GP must be to take full account of not only the presenting symptoms, the possible hidden agenda and the patient's underlying fears, but also to be able to empathize and ensure that the patient doesn't feel rushed (even though there may be a hundred other tasks to get done that morning with perhaps a potentially urgent visit to squeeze in). We must be able to offer advice and provide reassurance about the normal and benign while also having our minds fixed on the 'red-flag' danger signals. The balance between reassurance and cautionary investigation or referral can sometimes be extremely difficult. Therefore the GP has to develop skills that not only focus thoughts on clinical issues, but also help the patient to develop an understanding of their health problem, explore the patient's concerns and help them make informed decisions as to the best course of action.

Although each GP needs to develop their own style of consultation to meet these demands, there are some absolute requirements. Good listening skills and open questioning are essential. The only way to make your patient feel that they haven't been rushed and have been taken seriously is by listening properly to their problems and demonstrating a degree of empathy as to how they are feeling. Allowing your patient to express fully their symptoms and anxieties not only increases the likelihood of a correct diagnosis, but also usually leads to a more effective and often shorter consultation. In contrast, constantly interrupting with endless closed questions can frustrate your patient, prolong the consultation and mean that you miss vital verbal cues.

The other necessity is, of course, knowledge. Not only do you need the clinical knowledge to enable you to make an accurate diagnosis and treatment decision, but you also need to know about the local resources (e.g. counsellors, self-help groups) that might benefit your patient.

Sometimes it will be necessary to arrange a further consultation to work through your patient's presenting problems in more depth. When this is the case, it is useful to have part of the working week when this is most convenient, when there are fewer pressures on your time.

Examination skills

Examination skills need to be efficient and yet thorough. There is not enough time to complete an entire examination of even just one system, so the examination has to be focused to those clearly identified signs that may affect the actual management of the patient.

Interacting with colleagues

Interpersonal skills

Interpersonal skills certainly don't end with patient care. The ever-increasing trend towards teamwork and the closer ties between neighbouring practices with the

Interpersonal skills certainly **don't end** with patient care

advent of primary care groups/trusts mean that none of us can work in the isolation that has existed in the past. Success as a GP will increasingly depend on communication with colleagues as well as other professionals.

Teamwork and delegation

The framework of general practice is, as already mentioned, changing from hierarchy to teamwork, but the GP will maintain a pivotal role. We need to be able to work within the team, be central in developing the team and be able to delegate in a way that enhances safe patient care and ensures that we use our skills to the maximum benefit; we must realize that some problems are better addressed by others with better training and, perhaps, more time. We can't possibly know about everything and delegation, within the partnership, to a trusted and able practice manager as well as to the rest of the practice team, is essential in order to develop in the culture of efficient, effective and caring healthcare. The GP of the future needs, therefore, to be a leader but in a much less hierarchical system than has been typical in the past.

Good practice organization in primary care is a key to enjoyable and effective consultations with patients. Again, the exact arrangements will vary according to the needs and wishes of each individual doctor and practice, but effective methods for meeting patients' demands include:

- nurse triage of appointment requests
- adequate time for telephone consultations
- nurse practitioners
- open surgeries or one doctor rostered each day to deal with all urgent patient requests.

Many practices currently feel helpless against the tide of patient needs, but regular planning and improvement of practice organization can make enormous differences. An 'away day' is the ideal environment to set minds to these tasks, as long as the day itself is well planned and properly facilitated.

> Regular **improvement** of **practice organization** can make **enormous differences**

Audit of practice procedures is as important as audit of clinical management. Audit skills are now an absolute necessity for all doctors and nurses, and although audits can be seen as time-consuming, they can uncover surprising and invaluable information about the organization of the practice and can therefore help develop plans for improvement.

Guidelines and regulations

Evidence-based medicine and clinical governance

Although no one can deny the value of moving to evidence-based medicine and improved clinical governance, there is currently a very broad range of views as to the balance between the guideline-based approach and traditional individual-focused care. We are in a process of not only changing systems, but also of changing culture; this will see an increasing

Skills and attributes of a GP

understanding of the integration of these two principles of healthcare. This process is already well underway. It will be impossible to provide evidence for all our interventions, but all decisions and procedures need to be assessed in terms of benefit to the patient and cost-effectiveness, including the amount of time required for the process. Evidence-based practice has the potential to save time by avoiding interventions with no proven benefit, and should not be seen as just another drain on the little time available.

Avoiding information overload

The advent of the Internet gives health professionals, as well as patients, the potential to become infinitely more aware of research, guidelines, treatments and support groups. Although this provides enormous opportunities for improving healthcare, it raises the problem of information overload. We are in danger of receiving so many guidelines and protocols that each one gets filed and forgotten.

Computer technology itself can play a major role in overcoming these problems, with computer prompts and quick access to relevant information when required, but the successful GP will need to develop greater skills in critical appraisal.

The enormity of the information available doesn't necessarily imply that we need to know it all, just that we need to be able to access it when we need to. Learning should be based at a practical level. It is impossible to know everything about every condition, but it is essential to know the key aspects, including the appropriate interventions and when to refer. Learning from colleagues in primary and secondary care is often as effective as reading from books and Internet sources, and can provide much more practical information. Letters from consultants often provide a good learning tool, though their value is often overlooked.

> We just **need** to be able
> to **access information**
> when **required**

Putting guidelines into practice

Good communication and regular meetings between the clinical practice staff enable agreement to be reached and help generate the enthusiasm necessary to integrate new guidelines into clinical practice. Without this, the information, despite its quality and potential value, will not benefit us or our patients, becoming instead a hindrance to the implementation of good clinical practice.

There are two main essential requirements for implementing guidelines. The first is to understand them. It is impossible to remember guidelines if you don't fully understand the basis of the medical aspects of the condition and the evidence for the management options. An implication of this is that good critical appraisal skills are no longer optional, but mandatory.

> It is **vital** that **everyone** feels involved in the **guideline development** process

The second requirement is to involve and enthuse the rest of the practice team. All too often one or two members of the team feel isolated when trying to develop guidelines for the practice. It is vital that everyone feels involved in the development process or only half the practice will implement them, resulting in confusion for patients and poorer working relationships between the practice doctors and nurses.

Looking after yourself

General practice has always been a potentially stressful career and the need for a balanced lifestyle is becoming greater all the time. Reduced confidence of the public following successive high-profile scandals, as well as the pressures of increased expectations of primary care, make our job an extremely demanding, yet equally rewarding one. But we are only human, and have the same expectations and needs as everyone else. GPs must ensure that they do not lose the feelings of involvement and satisfaction with their career, even though they may feel that they are under attack from all directions. It is essential not to develop the nine-to-five mentality – time spent at evening meetings with colleagues can help to maintain the more positive feelings we have for general practice.

It is also good to have friends within the profession who can understand how we feel, particularly when specific difficulties, such as complaints, occur. But it is equally imperative to plan time as far away from medicine as possible. It is useful to have friends from a range of different occupations; becoming fixed on thinking and talking about work issues can become extremely destructive. To avoid excessive stress, make sure you spend time away from medicine from week to week, and plan (and take!) holidays where you escape from work completely.

> **Plan** (and take!) **holidays** where you **escape** from **work** completely

GPs are often guilty of not seeking help and support when they need it. We spend all day helping to analyse and resolve other people's problems, but don't have a clue when it comes to our own. There are now more and better avenues of support when problems do arise, and we must all be aware of them and make full use of all resources when necessary.

The key to being a successful GP, therefore, not only lies in clinical communication, interpersonal and critical appraisal skills, but most of all in understanding and accommodating our own fallibility and limitations.

training to be a GP

Dr John Toby, Chairman of the
Joint Committee on Postgraduate
Training for General Practice

Deciding to be a GP

The attraction of general practice

For many, the attraction of general practice
is its variety. There is variety within the
traditional surgery setting where the GP
never knows what sort of case he will be
dealing with next – a simple sore throat,
heart attack, schizophrenic breakdown,
pregnancy or a convulsing child. There is
variety in the type of work available to GPs
– they may work in the community, in
hospitals as occupational health physicians
and in more unusual settings, such as
mountain and sea rescue. They may work
for other organizations, such as the police,

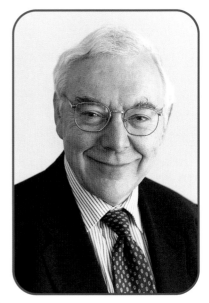

and as medical writers, advisers, teachers and trainers. The populations
they serve can range from the very deprived in inner cities and rural
areas to the more prosperous middle classes in towns and urban settings.
Finally, the type of practice can range from small, single-handed centres
to large health centres where the doctor works with a wide range of
other health professionals.

The GP's role

The core of the work of a GP is as a clinical generalist who is able to
understand the physical, psychological and social aspects of patients'

problems and make an initial assessment in all cases. In most cases, GPs are able to help patients in the management of their problems without reference to other agencies, but they also work closely with others in primary care and with specialist colleagues. Their training and experience therefore needs to be broad, but also sufficiently deep in specific areas to allow for the management of common problems wholly within primary care. Some GPs also have special interests that enable them to provide greater expertise in limited areas, either within primary care or in a hospital setting.

When to decide

Nearly half of those who qualify as doctors will become GPs. It is not necessary to decide between general practice or hospital medicine during medical school, because the educational programme for all is similar at undergraduate level. Medical education for all doctors increasingly involves primary care and some medical schools have particularly strong general practice departments.

> You don't have to **decide** between **general practice** or **hospital medicine** at medical school

Doctors who decide to train for general practice usually start training following successful completion of the pre-registration house officer year. Some decide they want to be GPs after some years in specialist medicine. The period of training for general practice is known as vocational or postgraduate training.

The training programme

The length and content of GP training is determined by parliamentary regulations[1] and is overseen by the Joint Committee on Postgraduate Training for General Practice (JCPTGP). Training is organized on a regional basis, however. Responsibility for the provision and organization of training within each deanery rests with the director of postgraduate GP education who is supported by a team of associate directors and course organizers. (Deaneries are geographical areas that correspond very roughly to old NHS regions and the spheres of interest of universities. The patterns have become rather blurred with time, but each deanery has a postgraduate dean, a director of postgraduate general practice education and one or more undergraduate deans.)

Training options

Trainees for general practice choose a formal 3-year vocational training scheme, construct their own programme from approved posts, or choose a mixture of both. Increasingly doctors are opting for formal schemes because they offer a better choice of posts specifically designed to prepare the trainee for this demanding profession.

Schemes are available throughout the UK. Doctors who choose a scheme have the security of knowing that their posts are arranged for the next 3 years. However, those who put together their own programme can include specialties in locations of their choosing (providing, of course, the posts are approved for GP training). Recruitment is coordinated centrally by each deanery. Schemes and individual posts are advertised bi-annually in the *BMJ*; GP trainers are no longer permitted to recruit directly to their own practices.

Full registration with the GMC is a prerequisite when applying for a scheme and GP registrar posts. Doctors who have limited registration may complete the hospital component of training, but must obtain full registration before applying for a GP registrarship.

Length of training

Regulations require 3 years of training. This has usually consisted of 24 months in Senior House Officer (SHO) posts and 12 months in general practice as a GP registrar. GP registrar posts are supernumerary. The regulations require at least 1 year of the training to be as a GP registrar and 1 year in hospital. Funding for more than 12 months as a GP registrar was not normally available until April 2000, when the budget for GP training passed to deaneries. It is now possible for a doctor to train as a GP registrar for more than 1 year, often in an innovative post with day release to other areas such as outpatient clinics. However, funds for these arrangements are limited.

Training can be split between different deaneries and posts undertaken in any order. It is generally accepted that the final phase of training should be as a GP registrar, so that hospital-based training can be seen in a general practice context and the chances of passing summative assessment maximized.

GP training can be undertaken on a part-time basis. For part-time training that began after 31 December 1994, the Regulations stipulate that training must be at least 60% of full time (i.e. a training programme that would take 3 years full-time would take 5 years part-time) and must also include at least two periods of full-time employment, each lasting not less than 1 week, with one being in hospital and one in general practice.[2]

Equivalent experience

Training that follows the standard format described is called 'prescribed experience', and will lead to the issue of a certificate of prescribed experience. Doctors whose training does not conform to the standard format, but consider it to be equivalent, can apply for a certificate of equivalent experience. Both certificates are valid for the purposes of entry into general practice and are of equal value.

> Prescribed and equivalent experience are equally valid

More details can be found in the JCPTGP guidance on the training programme and applying for a certificate.[3]

Re-training

Doctors who have not worked in general practice for some time and who are exempt from the need to have a JCPTGP certificate[4] can apply to their deanery for a period of funded familiarization training in a GP registrar post.

The JCPTGP

The JCPTGP, formed in 1976 from a partnership between the Royal College of General Practitioners (RCGP) and the General Practitioners' Committee

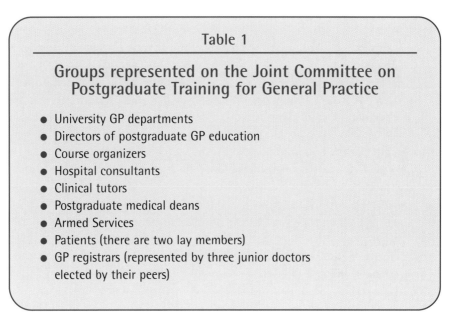

Table 1

Groups represented on the Joint Committee on Postgraduate Training for General Practice

- University GP departments
- Directors of postgraduate GP education
- Course organizers
- Hospital consultants
- Clinical tutors
- Postgraduate medical deans
- Armed Services
- Patients (there are two lay members)
- GP registrars (represented by three junior doctors elected by their peers)

of the BMA, comprises representatives from a number of groups (Table 1). The majority of members are working GPs.

Responsibilities

In general, the JCPTGP divides its time between issuing certificates of vocational training, setting the standards for GP education[5,6] and ensuring its quality through a system of visiting of deaneries (Table 2).[7] The selection of hospital posts and trainers, with their practices, is carried out on its behalf by deaneries and the RCGP.

At the time of writing, the arrangements for the supervision of medical education are being reviewed and the functions carried out by the JCPTGP may be undertaken within a different framework, but possibly in a similar way.

The hospital component of training

This has almost always been based on traditional senior house officer (SHO) posts although, in some schemes, some posts have been shortened

Table 2

Main responsibilities of the Joint Committee on Postgraduate Training for General Practice

- Setting the standards of GP training in the UK and Armed Services; this includes monitoring the performance of deaneries with regard to the provision of training programmes
- Approving posts for GP training
- Approving GP trainers
- Issuing certificates of prescribed and equivalent experience to doctors who have completed the training programme successfully
- Issuing certificates of acquired rights
- Acting as the Competent Authority in the UK for all the purposes of Title IV of Council Directive 93/16/EEC, which deals with arrangements for the training and employment of GPs in the European Economic Area (EEA)

and linked; for example, 12-months training might comprise up to three or four different posts. The regulations currently require two periods of 6 months from a shortlist of selected posts, with more freedom about the choice of remaining posts, provided they have been approved. While the results of the Government's current review of SHO posts remain to be announced, the principle of hospitals providing periods of training in a variety of specialties will be maintained.

The role of the trainer and the training practice

The time spent as a GP registrar is a very important part of the GP training programme. The JCPTGP and deaneries have criteria for the selection of trainers. Trainers are themselves trained to carry out their role and they are responsible for ensuring that other partners and members of the primary healthcare team contribute to the registrar's education. During their time in general practice, GP registrars must learn about the management of acute and long-term problems, preventive work and practice management. They must develop their own consulting and decision-making skills, learn to direct their own learning and acquire the ability to look critically at their own performance. It is the trainer's responsibility to enable the registrar to learn both within the practice and through attendance at local half-day release courses, visits to different types of practices and other local facilities.

The trainer is also responsible for making regular and documented formative assessments of the registrar's progress, and for assisting the registrar through the process of summative assessment and with the examination for membership of the RCGP.

Formative and summative assessment

Assessment has always been an important part of GP training.

Formative assessment

Formative assessment is used to measure progress at regular intervals so GP registrars can see how their training is progressing. Above all, formative assessment is for the benefit of the learner. It provides a record of progress at a given time, which is shared and discussed by registrar and trainer, and used to draw up a learning plan. Often registrars complete a logbook as part of this process. A wide variety of methods are used, including multiple-choice

> **Assessment is an important part of GP training**

questionnaires (MCQs), subjective and objective rating scales, consultation analysis (usually involving video recording), case analysis, feedback from patients, staff and colleagues, and other tools to identify learning needs.

Summative assessment

Summative assessment is a test of competence completed during or at the end of training, resulting in a pass or fail. It became mandatory by law in 1998 and serves a number of purposes, ensuring that patients are

---

Table 3

Competencies assessed in the summative assessment

- Factual medical knowledge sufficient to enable the practitioner to perform the duties of a GP
- The ability to apply factual medical knowledge to the management of problems presented by patients in general practice
- Effective communication, both orally and in writing
- The ability to consult satisfactorily with general practice patients
- The ability to review and analyse critically the practitioner's own working practices and manage any necessary changes appropriately
- Clinical skills
- The ability to synthesize all the above competencies and apply them appropriately in a general practice setting

---

provided with the protection of knowing that all doctors who complete GP training have had their competence assessed to a national standard. It also protects registrars by providing a route to any necessary extra training and lifts from trainers the burden of being the sole assessor. The standard is set at a constant level; there is no built-in failure rate. The vast majority of registrars have no difficulty passing.

The competencies tested are shown in Table 3. Four modules must be passed:

- MCQ
- assessment of consultation skills, using video or patient-simulated surgery
- written submission of practical work
- trainer's report.

A number of providers offer summative assessment tests and details can be obtained from the JCPTGP.

The MRCGP video is now an approved method for testing the consultation-skills component of summative assessment. To minimize work for the GP registrar, the RCGP and deaneries have set up a system in which the same tape can be submitted just once for both the examination leading to membership of the Royal College of General Practitioners (MRCGP) and summative assessment.[8]

Completion of training

Requirements

Each period of training that makes up the 3-year programme must be recorded using a statutory form confirming the total period of employment and whether it was completed to the satisfaction of the supervising doctor.

Posts that have not been approved for GP training may be considered under the regulatory provisions for equivalent experience. In these cases, a statement confirming the dates of employment and its satisfactory completion is required, as are a full job description and the recommendations of the local director as to the post's merits and relevance to GP training.

Training outside the UK

Doctors who have trained outside the UK in another European Economic Area (EEA) country should complete an application form for equivalent experience and special forms for hospital posts held within the EEA. Doctors who have trained overseas – outside the EEA – also need to complete an application form as well as special forms for hospital posts held overseas.

> Each period of training must be officially recorded

Doctors who have a medical degree from a university within the EEA and whose training was completed under the supervision of the JCPTGP are entitled to practise throughout Europe. If their medical degree or any part of their postgraduate training was completed outside the EEA, they are not automatically qualified to practise throughout Europe. If, however, they have a certificate from the JCPTGP, they are able to practise within the UK. Under current regulations the certificate is not time barred and once issued may be used any time in the future. If the JCPTGP refuses to issue a certificate, the applicant has a statutory right of appeal to the Secretaries of State for Health.

The MRCGP

The MRCGP was introduced in 1965. It was not then, and is not now, a compulsory part of GP registrar training. However, it is recognized as the 'gold standard' assessment method for GP registrars, and some partnerships will only appoint GPs with the MRCGP. The examination is a test of:
- clinical knowledge and diagnostic skills
- consulting and communication skills
- practice management
- attitudes in areas such as ethics and medical politics.

Since 1998, the MRCGP has been a credit-accumulation examination in which modules can be taken at the same session, or different sessions and in any order over a 3-year period. There are four modules: paper 1, paper 2, an oral examination and a test of consulting skills.

Tips for getting the most out of your training

- Make use of all the practice and primary care teams in your local area to help your training. The practice nurses and manager can be very good sources of information on a variety of key topics.
- Start practising making videos early on in your GP registrar year. Ensure that the video that you finally submit is technically sound. Some videos are rejected because of poor sound or picture quality.
- Take the summative assessment MCQ early to get it over and done with – you can take it as many times as you wish, but if you fail twice you are likely to be called to the deanery to discuss your training and progress in general.
- Remember that the MRCGP MCQ and video are both accepted components of summative assessment – kill two birds with one stone by opting for these methods.
- Keep your summative assessment audit simple. You are aiming to show that you understand the principles of audit, not that you

have carried out an audit that has fundamentally changed the way your practice operates.

- Always end the training programme with a period of at least 6 months as a GP registrar, rather than in a hospital post. This will enable you to see your hospital training in a general practice context, and will maximize the chance of success in summative assessment.
- Ask the JCPTGP to check the completeness of your hospital programme in advance of making a formal application for a certificate (i.e. submit all but your final VTR form during your last post). Again, this will minimize the chance of delays in the issuing of your certificate. If you have unusual UK, EEA or overseas experience, you are strongly advised to approach the Joint Committee for an assessment of your experience some time before making your formal application; the verification of overseas experience and the Committee's assessment of it can take some time – up to 3 months.
- The JCPTGP will accept formal applications for certificates up to 1 month before completion of the final training post – if you apply early there is much less chance that your starting date will be delayed. Remember that doctors cannot work in **any** capacity in general practice until they are in possession of a Joint Committee certificate.

Website and address

The JCPTGP's website is at http://www.jcptgp.org.uk.
The Committee can also be contacted at its registered offices:
14 Princes Gate
London SW7 1PU

References

1   NHS (Vocational Training for General Medical Practice) Regulations 1997. Statutory Instrument no. 2817 (England and Wales) and corresponding regulations for Scotland and Northern Ireland.

2.   *Guidelines on part time (flexible) training.* London: JCPTGP, 1998.

3.   *A Guide to Certification.* London: JCPTGP, 2001.

4.   *A Guide to Certification.* London: JCPTGP, 2001: chapter 12.

5.   *Recommendations to Deaneries on the Selection and Re-Selection of General Practice Trainers.* London: JCPTGP, 2001.

6.   *Recommendations on the Selection and Re-Selection of Hospital Posts for General Practice Training.* London: JCPTGP, 2001.

7.   *A Guide to Accreditation Visits.* London: JCPTGP, 2001.

8.   Field S. *The Single Route to Assessment of Consultation Skills.* Fact Sheet, September 2000.

Further reading

Ferguson JF. *MRCGP Preparation and Passing.* London: The Royal Society of Medicine Press, 2000.

Membership of the Royal College of General Practitioners. RCGP Information Sheet (July). London: RCGP, 1999.

choosing a practice

Dr Tony Stanton, Secretary to the London
Local Medical Committees

General practice is moving into a new era in which what was historically a single way to provide NHS general practice is changing into a mixed economy. So what are the choices open to aspiring GPs?

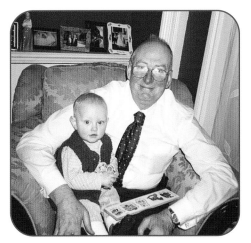

Independent contractor status

The main way of practising as a GP is still as an independent contractor. Unlike doctors employed by hospitals and community trusts, most GPs operate as independent contractors – they are self-employed and have entered into arrangements with a health authority to provide general medical services (GMS). This arrangement is provided for in Part 2 of the NHS Act, which previously specifically prohibited the remuneration of those doctors by means of a fixed salary other than in very special and limited circumstances. This requirement was ended by the Health and Social Care Act 2001.

> **Most GPs** operate as **independent contractors**

The way in which health authorities are required to implement these arrangements is laid down in very great detail in a set of regulations (the NHS General Medical Services Regulations, 1992) that are quite frequently amended. Those regulations require health authorities to pay fees and allowances and to reimburse many practice expenses on the basis of the Statement of Fees and Allowances, almost universally known as 'the Red Book'. The actual amounts of those fees and allowances are specified each year by the Doctor's and Dentist's Review Body.

Terms of service

What perhaps might be termed the 'job description' of a GP is, in effect, laid down in a schedule to the NHS Regulations called the Terms of Service for Doctors, which specifies in very great detail what a GP must and must not do. Strictly speaking, therefore, there is no such thing as a contract for independent contractors providing GMS, but there is this set of fairly detailed arrangements, all of which are negotiated centrally by the BMA's General Practitioners' Committee; many elements of their local implementation require consultation with the Local Medical Committee (LMC).

Options as an independent contractor

Doctors wanting to work as independent contractors have two ways in which they may do so. They may:
- apply for a nationally advertised sole practitioner vacancy
- apply to join another GP or GPs in partnership.

Sole practitioner
Sole practitioner vacancies are advertised by health authorities, usually in the *BMJ*. They nearly always occur as a replacement for a previous sole practitioner, so normally there is an established list of patients. However, premises occupied by the previous doctor may no longer be available and, as an independent contractor, it is the responsibility of the successful applicant to provide their own premises, staff and computers. Help may well be available from the health authority (or its successor) and from the local primary care organization, but seeking to establish yourself as a

> Seeking to **establish** yourself **as** a **sole practitioner** is a substantial **challenge**

Table 1

Advantages and disadvantages of independent contractor status

Advantages

- Nationally negotiated and priced contractual arrangements
- High level of job security until compulsory retirement at 70 years of age
- Working under a tried and tested system with a considerable element of flexibility

Disadvantages

- Being personally responsible for ensuring the provision of care to your patients
- A certain amount of frustrating bureaucracy
- A complicated remuneration system that does not always yield the headline pay awards recommended by the Review Body

sole practitioner is a substantial challenge. You will be expected to demonstrate a business plan.

Established partnerships

Most doctors join established partnerships, either as a replacement partner or as an additional partner. Sole practitioners are required to have full-time availability, though this requirement can be met by working in a job-share arrangement. Partnership vacancies can be for full-time, three-quarter-time or half-time availability. Again, full-time vacancies can be delivered by a job-share arrangement, though this does not apply to three-quarter- or half-time vacancies.

Advantages and disadvantages

The advantages and disadvantages of independent contractor status are listed in Table 1.

Personal medical services

Personal medical services (PMS) are currently operated as pilots under the provisions of the Primary Care Act 1997. Essentially, this Act permits the provision of traditional GP services by what are termed NHS bodies as opposed to individual GPs. Pilot bodies may be:

- existing practices or groups of practices (the majority)
- already established NHS Trusts, usually community trusts
- new NHS bodies created for the purpose (e.g. nurse-led pilots).

In broad terms, PMS pilots have to provide the same sort of patient services as are required under GMS, but they may also choose to bid to provide additional services. It is a common fallacy that PMS pilots equate to a salaried service – most PMS pilots consist of GPs who have switched from their GMS arrangements, and who remain independent contractors.

Table 2

The advantages and disadvantages of personal medical services pilots

Advantages

- Encourage innovation and flexibility
- Ability to agree the contract price for the pilot locally
- Opportunity to attract additional funding to employ extra doctors and nurse practitioners
- Regular and equal monthly payments of one-twelfth of the contract price

Disadvantages

- Difficult to negotiate in-year contract variations
- Annual reviews of the contract content and its pricing
- Contract price becoming part of the unified budget of the primary care team/health authority and therefore subject to the same constraints as the rest of that budget

---

Salaried options are discussed in the next section. The advantages and disadvantages of PMS pilots are given in Table 2.

With each wave of PMS pilots, the contractual arrangements have become much more detailed and there is now a national core contract, as well as detailed directions to health authorities that closely mimic the GMS regulations.

Salaried options

Doctors looking for a salaried option have the following choices. They can work:

- as an assistant to a GMS independent contractor
- as a salaried doctor employed by a PMS pilot, the employer being:
  - a PMS pilot partnership
  - a Trust
  - a nurse-led pilot.

Whichever one of these options you choose, it is vital to ensure that you have a proper job description and a robust contract of employment; BMA members may obtain expert advice from BMA Regional Offices.

Principal or non-principal?

Doctors who choose to work as independent GMS contractors or who join PMS pilots as a partner can probably equally be regarded as principals.

Doctors not wishing to make such a commitment may choose to work as a non-principal, which is a generic term for doctors who deputize for GP principals, whether as assistants, locums, or retainees. This can be a very useful way of gaining experience in a range of different

> **Working** as a **non-principal** can be a **useful** way of **gaining experience**

practices and can also fit in with other commitments such as other professional activities, family commitments or additional interests. The BMA's General Practitioners' Committee has published guidance on the retainer scheme and on contracts for assistants.

Practice agreements

Practice agreements are the normal way of underpinning partnership arrangements. There are many different types of partnership, ranging from an informal association between two or more GPs, without any express partnership agreement, through to elaborate agreements, sometimes including sophisticated management structures. The information in Table 3 has been extracted from guidance prepared by the BMA's General Practitioners' Committee.

A doctor joining an existing partnership, even for a period of mutual assessment, means that a new legal partnership has been created. If either a new partnership agreement or a supplementary deed is not fully in place before the new doctor joins the practice, then a 'partnership at will' exists which has a number of consequences attached (Table 3).

If the existing partnership cannot produce a copy of an up-to-date agreement or, even more worryingly, states that there is one but they cannot find it, then warning bells should ring. The bells should be even louder if the incoming doctor is refused access to the practice accounts or obstacles are put in the way of seeking accountancy or legal advice.

Pitfalls on entering practice

Pitfalls are many and varied and, although not all can be predicted, they tend to concern the five Ps:

- profits
- property
- patients
- performance
- personalities.

Profits

There should be no shame in highlighting the issue of practice profits since a key definition of partnership is two or more people working together precisely with that aim in life. It is therefore absolutely crucial to establish from the outset precisely what should be included as partnership income, what should be counted as practice expenses and what as

Table 3

Why have a partnership agreement?

- Partnership disputes are common. Although a properly drafted partnership agreement may not prevent disputes, it may lessen their impact or avoid them altogether
- A partnership without an up-to-date written agreement is a 'partnership at will', meaning that relations between partners are governed by the Partnership Act 1890. A 'partnership at will' is the most unstable business relationship that exists as it can be dissolved at any time with the following consequences:
  - notice may be served by any one partner on the others without their prior knowledge or consent
  - it may take immediate effect and no reason need be given to justify it
  - it may result in the forced sale of all partnership assets (including the surgery premises) and the redundancy of all staff
  - there is nothing to prevent any one partner, or group of partners, from immediately forming a new practice/partnership to the exclusion of the other partner(s)
  - there is no deemed restrictive covenant*
- During the lifetime of a 'partnership at will', all partners are deemed to have equal profit shares unless there is clear evidence to the contrary, and most decisions may be made by simple majority. Thus, a written agreement should reduce significantly the potential for serious disagreements and instability

*Restrictive covenants seek to limit the ability of a partner who is leaving the practice from working as a GP within a defined area for a fixed period of time. The limitations have to be reasonable in order to be enforceable.

personal expenses, so that all parties have a clear understanding of how the profits of the practice are calculated. A clear agreement about sharing profits (or indeed losses) is vital, together with a clear schedule and timetable of profit shares to parity.

Property

All practices own property, for example equipment, surgery fittings and furniture, and agreement is needed as to how and when a new partner buys into those assets. In addition, all practices occupy surgery premises and the basis of their ownership or lease arrangements must be absolutely clear. Particular attention must be paid to avoiding the pitfall of any concealed sale of goodwill.

Patients

A fair and equitable share of patient registrations should be the ideal, and any patient should be entitled to register with any partner in the practice, subject only to that partner's agreement.

Performance

Division of work and clinical performance are frequent causes of dissension within partnerships. The commitment of each partner should be clearly stated within the partnership agreement and the practice needs to have robust clinical governance arrangements.

Personalities

Not even the best partnership agreement can save doctors from problems of conflicting personalities. A decent period of mutual assessment (at least 6 months – arguably 12) will at least provide an opportunity for the prospective new partner and the existing partners to see whether they really can work together. If it does not feel right, it is probably best for everyone if problems are faced up to at an early stage and, if they cannot be resolved, it may well be better to go for a clean break than to endure years of pain.

being a GP

Dr Chris Nancollas, GP

Delivery of general or PMS

Once you have decided which type of practice or organization you wish to join, the next step is to consider what exactly you will be doing. 'General practice' is a nebulous phrase that conceals a number of quite specific tasks, from dealing with the acute and chronic manifestations of disease, to maternity, child health and disease prevention

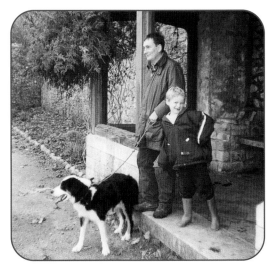

(Table 1). You'll need to keep up to date with advances in medicine, apply national service frameworks and keep an eye on both your own and your colleagues' practice. In order to do this, you will need to be part of an efficient organization, which will require you to master the complexities of finance, management and information technology. As well as all this, you will be working in a system where the demands for your time far outstrip the supply.

> **No one** can master the **skills necessary** for **success** in **all** the **disciplines** of **general practice**

It sounds daunting, and it is, but you need to remember one thing. No one can master the skills necessary to achieve success in all the disciplines of general practice. What you need are three qualities:

Table 1

Delivering general medical services

Clinical

Acute medicine
- Emergencies 0700 hours – 1900 hours
- Out of hours

Chronic medicine
- Disease management protocols
- National service frameworks
- NICE guidelines

Others
- Maternity
- Child health
- Preventive medicine

External clinical commitments
- Clinical assistantships
- Occupational health

Managerial
- Staff
- Premises
- Finance
- Computer
- Formulary
- Practice development plan
- Patient liaison

Educational
- Personal development plans
- Clinical governance
- Clinical meetings
- Developing protocols and guidelines

Political
- Local medical committee work
- Primary care group work

- honesty, or the ability to identify your strengths and weaknesses
- organization, in order to make the best of your time
- tough-mindedness – the ability to say 'no'.

The last bullet point may sound peculiar, but it is the most valuable and, needless to say, the most difficult skill to acquire.

Teamwork

As well as having the requisite personal qualities, the successful GP will be one who is part of a good team. The key point here is an understanding of teamwork, and how different types of people bring different qualities to the team.

Ask yourself:

- am I happy with the way we make decisions?
- do we follow these through?
- can we manage conflict?

> Nothing **fragments** a **partnership** quicker than dysfunctional management

These and other questions may sound obtuse, but they will soon become part of your daily life. If the answers to any or all of them is 'no', then it is time to reappraise the way you make decisions. Nothing fragments a partnership quicker than dysfunctional management.

Out-of-hours work and responsibility

Out-of-hours work is the single most unpopular part of the GP contract. You are working when you are tired, the patients are demanding, cases come along in unmanageable clumps, and it is fertile ground for complaints. I mention this not to frighten you, but to reassure you that you are not alone.

The situation has improved in recent years with the expansion of commercial deputizing services and the creation of GP cooperatives. If you are a principal you must remember that you are still technically responsible for your patients, so you must satisfy yourself that your deputies are competent. Commercial deputizing services will be responsible for this 'in-house', but GP cooperatives are required to demonstrate that they review and monitor the service they offer. This means practising audit and clinical governance, and having a robust system for dealing with complaints.

Non-core clinical activities

Many practices build into their system time to pursue other interests like clinical assistantships, factory work, or school medicals. These perform two useful functions. They give you a break from the often frenetic pace of practice life, and they can be a valuable source of extra income.

Access to GPs

Contrary to popular opinion, access to British GPs is actually quite reasonable, given the structure and financing of the NHS. It is worth remembering that the public ideal – an appointment when it's wanted for as long as it's wanted – is unattainable, and we have to deal with the art of the possible.

Most practices will offer some sort of 'same-day' emergency service, and many doctors find that being available at some time of the day to make or receive phone calls saves a lot of work. There's little doubt that the successful GP of the future will also have to master effective communication with patients via the Internet and e-mail, as these will play an increasingly important role in the management of disease.

The most important person involved in accessing the GPs is the receptionist, so this can be a good test of practice teamwork and communication. It is important that your receptionists understand how the practice works, and the limits and responsibilities of their role. A properly trained and efficient receptionist makes your job so much easier.

And don't forget to look at your practice from a patient's point of view – ask yourself if you would be happy with the service.

Running an appointment system

Running an appointment system, which seems a simple matter of dividing consultations by doctors, is, in fact, fiendishly difficult. The main reason for this is that no two doctors work in the same way. Some are time-oriented, while others are habitually late. Some can see high numbers of patients very quickly, others find this impossible, and so on. Add to this the fact that every GP is privately convinced that he or she is the only one in the practice doing any work, and you have a potentially volatile situation.

The situation is further complicated by the fact that consultations are becoming more complex as we get loaded down with guidelines and frameworks. No one can be definitive about appointments, but I offer the following suggestions:

- the majority of routine appointments should be 10 minutes
- seeing high numbers of patients, 20–30+, during every surgery is extremely taxing
- there is a limit to the length of time you can consult.

At the time of writing, the Government is keen that routine appointments are available within 48 hours. Most practices struggle to offer them within 3–5 days.

Seeing urgent patients

Every practice needs to have a system for seeing 'urgent' patients. A good definition of urgent is 'a problem that cannot be safely left until the next routine appointment'. How you manage them varies widely. Some practices have an 'on-call' doctor, others have an open-access or single-problem surgery, while some just fit them in around routine work.

> Every practice needs a system for seeing urgent patients

Whatever system you choose, it is important to ensure it is not abused. Some kind of triage is probably essential, as is the need to develop a practice approach to those who misuse the system.

Controlling demand and your workload

Not so long ago, every patient who presented to a practice would be seen by a doctor. With the expansion of the role of practice nurses, and the concept of team working, that idea is now outmoded; in fact, the doctor who tries to do everything today will rapidly become overloaded. Table 2 highlights the range of expertise available.

The practice needs to consider ways, where possible, of controlling demand. The following questions may be useful:

- Does the patient need to come to the practice, or would telephone advice suffice?
- Does the patient need to see a doctor, or would seeing another member of the primary care team be more appropriate?
- Is the service the patient is asking for appropriate (for example, is an ambulant patient asking for a home visit)?
- Is the patient requesting the right doctor?

Regarding this last point, some patients with complex illnesses present to one doctor for the initial consultation, and then another for the

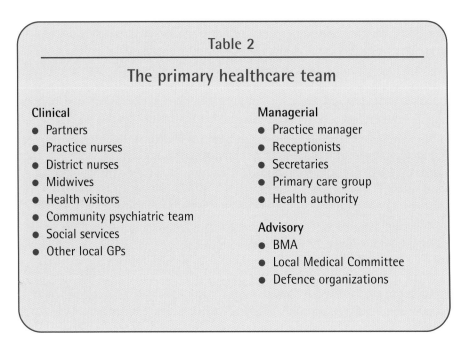

Table 2

The primary healthcare team

Clinical
- Partners
- Practice nurses
- District nurses
- Midwives
- Health visitors
- Community psychiatric team
- Social services
- Other local GPs

Managerial
- Practice manager
- Receptionists
- Secretaries
- Primary care group
- Health authority

Advisory
- BMA
- Local Medical Committee
- Defence organizations

results of investigations such as blood tests; this is frustrating for the doctors concerned, and potentially harmful to the patient. There are two ways of dealing with this, either by operating a personal list system, or by drawing up a contract with the patient whereby they agree to follow certain rules.

Clinically, there is often not much room for manoeuvre. Administratively, there is. Far too many doctors are wasting time doing things that another member of the practice team could do better, like inputting data on the computer, chasing up smears, or summarizing notes. The successful doctor is always asking himself or herself 'Do I really need to be doing this?' You'll be pleasantly surprised at the range of expertise in the practice team if you only ask.

> Too much **time** is **wasted** doing things that **another** member of the practice team could **do better**

I hope some or all of this will be useful to you. Remember that the successful GP is not necessarily the one who performs these tasks best, but the one who enjoys them most.

Useful websites

These include:
British Medical Journal at www.bmj.com
Royal College of General Practitioners at www.rcgp.org.uk
(this site has a particularly good section on access)

Further reading

The literature is vast, but a good overview of general practice is provided by the Oxford General Practice series (Oxford Medical Publications).

Selected other titles include:

Blanchard K, Johnson S. *The One Minute Manager*. London: HarperCollins, 1996.

Briggs Myers I. *Introduction to Type*. Oxford: Oxford Psychologists Press, 1998.

Department of Health. *Statement of Fees and Allowances* (the 'Red Book'). London: DoH, 1996.

Department of Health. *Personal Medical Service Pilots Under the NHS (Primary Care) Act*. London: DoH, 1997.

General Medical Council. *Good Medical Practice*. London: GMC, 1998.

General Medical Council. *Maintaining Good Medical Practice*. London: GMC, 1998.

hazards in practice

Dr Brian Goss, GP and Chairman,
Suffolk Local Medical Committees

Complaints from patients or relatives

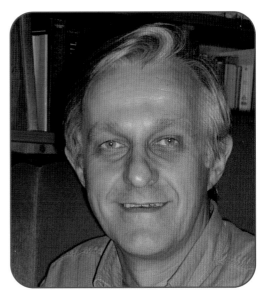

Most doctors try their best for patients, often in difficult circumstances. They entered the profession to help people, and are always hurt and upset by complaints about their performance. Politicians, the media and the appalling behaviour of a few of our colleagues seem to be conspiring to sap patients' confidence in doctors generally. Complaints to the GMC are rising at a rate of 30–50%/year.

The solution may seem to be to find another job, but actually the majority of patient complaints in general practice are understandable and can be resolved with either an explanation or a change in practice procedures. As a profession we need to be less tender about complaints and more ready to see them as a constructive part of practice life.

The heart of complaint management is an effective informal procedure, as required by the terms of service or PMS contract. The practice manager or deputy should take details of verbal complaints and respond immediately to written ones, indicating that a doctor not involved in the case will investigate and report to the complainant. In the process, ensure that the consent of the patient has been sought when the patient is an adult.

Obtain written reports from anyone involved. On the basis of the complaint and the reports you should be able to put most complaints into one of the following categories, which will determine how you should respond. In roughly descending order of frequency, you are likely to find the following causes in a good practice.

- Correct clinical care and handling – explain why what was done was correct even though it may have appeared wrong or had a poor outcome.
- Correct care but human error (including rudeness) within it – acknowledge, apologize and, if feasible, indicate any safety or preventive measure that can be built in.
- Unsafe system or poor practice – acknowledge, apologize and explain how you have changed the system so that it is safe and changed the practice or the practitioner if performance is poor.

Where possible, I like to see the complainant in person when I have investigated the complaint so that he or she has the opportunity of questioning me about my explanation. This also gives the opportunity for the complainant to see, from the time I have set aside and my willingness to listen, that I am taking their complaint seriously and seeking to learn from it rather than simply dismissing it out of hand.

> Most **complaints** are **understandable** and can be **resolved** with either an **explanation** or a **change** in **procedures**

After the interview, write to the complainant summarizing the meeting and offering a further opportunity for queries. If you think this is time-consuming, it is, but the time and distress to the doctor pales to insignificance compared with the anxiety of defending groundless complaints through formal channels. If a second meeting fails to resolve the problem or the complainant remains dissatisfied with the informal procedure, you must refer them to the health authority.

Very few complaints proceed beyond the informal stage, and details of the progression are beyond the scope of this book. However, with any serious complaint that is likely to proceed, or with a vexatious complainant, you should seek early advice from your medical protection organization.

Violent patients

Staff and doctors should be trained in prevention. Recognition of aggressive body language, having systems to minimize waiting and frustration, and being prepared to act to defuse developing situations are all essential.

Have clear systems for calling the police at the first sign of trouble. The mere presence of a police officer around the building often defuses a situation without him or her having to take any action. Where there is actual assault or frightening verbal abuse, the police should always be called, a complaint should be pressed formally and an incident number obtained.

> Have **clear systems** for calling the **police** at the first sign of **trouble**

Paragraph 9a of the Terms of Service permits the immediate removal of violent and abusive patients from a GP's list, but only after the police have been called and an incident number has been allocated. It is important for the prevention of violence that a zero tolerance policy is adopted consistently. The health authority will then allocate violent patients to properly set-up facilities where challenging behaviour can be dealt with appropriately. The crown prosecution service and the courts are also guided by government policy to view assaults on health service staff as the serious threat to society generally that they are.

Sometimes it will be necessary to consider injunctions after an episode of violence. If, for any reason the offender does not receive a custodial sentence, you may be justifiably concerned about treating the household contacts (usually women and children) of the (usually male) assailant. If these patients are not also allocated to the special arrangements, consider taking out an injunction restraining the offender from approaching your surgery or from being present in or near the residence when a house call has been requested. Breach of an injunction is an arrestable offence and is treated as contempt of court. Your practice solicitor can advise on taking out an injunction, and some health authorities may be prepared to assist with the legal costs in recognition of your willingness to continue to assist in these difficult circumstances.

Other reasons for removing patients from the list

There is usually only public sympathy when patients are removed from GPs' lists for violence. Removal for other reasons can attract unwelcome publicity. The patients usually present themselves as blameless and claim that their first inkling of a problem in an otherwise blissful doctor–patient relationship was the removal notice. Having investigated a number of cases, I have found that in the overwhelming majority of cases, there was a long history of unreasonable, abusive and aggressive patient behaviour, eventually causing the GP's patience to snap. The final straw on the camel's back is often not terribly heavy. But it is the straw and not the load that gets the publicity. This can be prevented.

In the face of unreasonable behaviour that falls short of violence or abuse, use your informal complaints procedure to register a complaint against the patient. Write to the patient detailing the behaviour and invite him or her to come and discuss it. There is no need to mention removal at this stage because, in my experience, the patient does not usually turn up to the meeting but the behaviour stops or the patient voluntarily registers elsewhere.

If the behaviour persists, send a further letter regretting the behaviour and indicating that you intend to remove the patient in the event of a recurrence. If you then need to ask for removal, there can be no question that the patient could have thought that all was well with their doctor. (See also page 49 on dealing with the press.)

Partnership problems

Like marriage, partnership can be an abiding joy or an unfolding nightmare. Always remember the wise words of Roger Neighbour – "If you don't think you're doing more than your partners, you're not doing as much". To which I often add "and if your spouse doesn't think you're doing more than your share, your partners are probably planning to expel you".

The division of workload and money are the two most common causes of partnership disharmony. Financial disagreements can often be prevented by a fair and well-drafted partnership agreement, but workload is more problematic. Do you equate time in the practice, consultation numbers and patient numbers? How do you allow for age, sex and morbidity structure and the effects of part-time versus whole-time working?

Sadly, there is no simple formula, and in the end individual practices and doctors must take a view on what is fair. Always be prepared to consider that it may be you that is wrong, or you that is not pulling your weight, and never rely on a single statistical analysis. Only when all the analyses point to the same answer is it possible to draw conclusions. Otherwise you may be best asking yourself whether you are happy overall. If you are, it is probably as much of a waste of time to try to define practice workload as to define art or beauty. If you are not happy, perhaps it is time to move on, whatever the numbers say.

> Like marriage, partnership can be an abiding joy or an unfolding nightmare

Always remember, though, that you are a partner and not an employee, and in particular that your partners are not your employers. So you cannot look to your partners to provide the cover or the finance needed to ensure the comfort, income, overtime pay, maternity rights or sick leave that you would be entitled to if you were an employee. If you don't like that statement, perhaps you should be looking for salaried employment.

Finally, two golden rules. First, if possible, keep the lawyers poor by conciliation and constructive negotiation. Secondly, never involve patients or the GMC in a partnership squabble – doing either places you at risk of an unwelcome appearance before a conduct committee even if you started as the complainant. Reserve the GMC for those cases where poor performance or behaviour places patients at risk, when you are obliged to take steps to protect patients.

Sexual harassment

Sexual harassment is unacceptable however it occurs and must be confronted early. However it is important to establish the facts clearly. There should be a well-understood and simple policy banning the early stages of harassment. For example, forbidding uninvited personal remarks even of a positive nature may assist by placing a disciplinary tripwire in the way of more inappropriate behaviour (Table 1).

Table 1

Actions that may constitute sexual harassment*

- Unwanted physical contact
- Demands for sexual favours in return for promotion
- Unwelcome sexual advances or propositions
- Continued offers of social contact outside the workplace when these have previously been rejected
- Offensive flirtations
- Suggestive remarks, innuendo or lewd comments
- Display of sexually suggestive pictures
- Leering
- Derogatory remarks that are gender-related
- Sexual assault
- Offensive comments about appearance or dress that are gender-related
- Sexist or patronizing behaviour

*Adapted with permission from Ellis N, 1998.

Sexual harassment is a variant of sexual offending, and will either respond promptly to confrontation or will prove intractable – as sexual offending is generally.

Be prepared to take early and firm action if early confrontation fails. If patients are victims, the GMC will need to be involved.

More detail on this subject, and racial or sexual discrimination, as well as all aspects of your obligations as an employer can be found in Norman Ellis's excellent *General Practice Employment Handbook*.

Racial or sexual discrimination

The Race Relations and Sex Discrimination Acts now apply to the smallest of employers. It is not sufficient to think that because you believe that you harbour no personal prejudice and have no intention to discriminate that you will automatically comply with the law.

Employers must act (and, importantly, be able to show that they have acted) without discrimination, so your procedures should be demonstrably fair, and your criteria for shortlisting and appointment explicit and defensible. Also, beware of indirect discrimination, which can occur for example if unreasonable educational requirements are stipulated for a menial post. Perhaps the most common potential for unintentional discrimination lies with the handling of applications from men for receptionist posts.

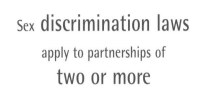

Sex **discrimination laws** apply to partnerships of **two or more**

Although appointing partners is not an employment matter, sex discrimination laws apply to partnerships of two or more and race discrimination where there are five or more. However, discrimination is a GMC offence whatever numbers are involved.

Dealing with the media after a crisis

You are only likely to have to deal with the media under two circumstances. First, you or a colleague may have done something shockingly wrong and have been found out. Second, a vindictive complainant has gone to the media before going through the proper complaint and/or legal procedures in order to embarrass you and obtain redress – often because they realize that their substantive case is weak.

As soon as you get wind of media involvement, decide rapidly with advice from colleagues and your defence organization which category you are in and act accordingly. The approaches are different. You will either need to 'admit and apologize', or 'rebut and explain'.

Admit and apologize

The lesson of Watergate is forgotten time and time again, but you should remember it. More people can remember the slow and evasive exposure of the truth than what Richard Nixon actually did wrong. However badly someone has behaved, a prompt full and frank admission with a sincere apology (covering not only what has been discovered but what could be discovered) is only 1 day's news and will be a stale story by tomorrow morning. Journalists love nothing better than to uncover a story a piece at a time so that each little detail gets a day's coverage. Fifty wrongdoings uncovered one at a time is 50 days' news. Fifty wrongdoings uncovered on 1 day is 1 day's news.

Rebut and explain

Doctors usually feel hamstrung by confidentiality when they are suddenly pitched into defending themselves outside the usual complaints or legal procedures. Remember that journalists have ethical codes too, and they are required to seek both sides of a story. Rather than try to shelter behind 'No comment', which is interpreted as an admission of guilt, consider instead saying 'I will be very happy to comment, but you will understand that I will need the written consent of all patients involved to divulge confidential information from their medical record in order to give my side of the story. If you would like to come back to me with that written consent, I shall be pleased to comment.'

> **Doctors** usually feel **hamstrung** by **confidentiality**

This approach, I should say, runs counter to the usual 'No comment' advice of the defence bodies. However, it has been used by a number of doctors who I have assisted with publicity arising from removals from their lists, and in all cases the journalists have dropped the story for lack of consent. In my experience, in the majority of patient-removal cases, the doctors have been saintly models of patience. The last thing the removed patient wants is the catalogue of their abuse of the NHS and its staff reaching the newspapers. What they wanted was an unrestrained go at the doctor, who would look guilty with 'no comment'. No responsible journalist will publish a story where the

> **Journalists rarely misquote,** although they often **quote selectively**

complainant uses legal or other means to prevent the other side dealing fully with the allegations.

Journalists are much maligned, but in nearly 20 years of dealing with them I have found that they rarely misquote, although they often quote selectively, and they usually seek a balanced story if all parties are prepared to respond promptly. Some tips for dealing with the media are given in Table 2, and BMA members can obtain help from the BMA Public Affairs Division in connection with individual cases.

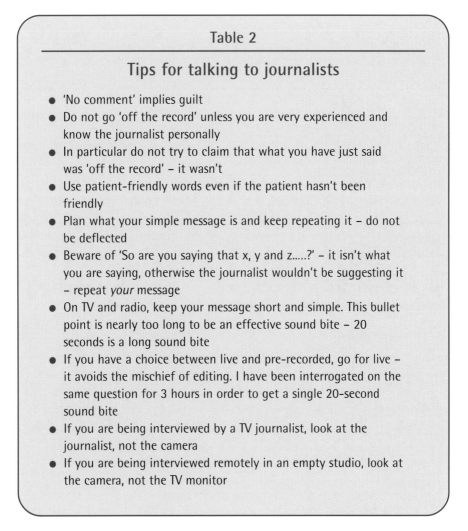

Table 2

Tips for talking to journalists

- 'No comment' implies guilt
- Do not go 'off the record' unless you are very experienced and know the journalist personally
- In particular do not try to claim that what you have just said was 'off the record' – it wasn't
- Use patient-friendly words even if the patient hasn't been friendly
- Plan what your simple message is and keep repeating it – do not be deflected
- Beware of 'So are you saying that x, y and z.....?' – it isn't what you are saying, otherwise the journalist wouldn't be suggesting it – repeat *your* message
- On TV and radio, keep your message short and simple. This bullet point is nearly too long to be an effective sound bite – 20 seconds is a long sound bite
- If you have a choice between live and pre-recorded, go for live – it avoids the mischief of editing. I have been interrogated on the same question for 3 hours in order to get a single 20-second sound bite
- If you are being interviewed by a TV journalist, look at the journalist, not the camera
- If you are being interviewed remotely in an empty studio, look at the camera, not the TV monitor

Further reading

Ellis N. *General Practice Employment Handbook*. Abingdon: Radcliffe Medical Press, 1998.

Neighbour R. *The Inner Consultation*. Reading: Petroc Press, 1987.

effective communication

Dr Kathryn Greaves, Assistant Director,
Medical Education Unit,
University of Aberdeen

Skilful communication is an essential component of medical practice. The skills required will vary according to the person with whom you are dealing – a patient or a colleague – and the particular circumstance.

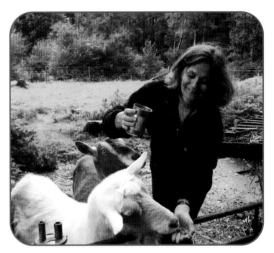

Talking to your patients

Most patients prefer to consult a practitioner who practises the 'art' of medicine in addition to being proficient in the 'science' of the subject. The discovery of a personal illness is bad enough, but it is worse to have to justify your worries under pressure of time to a brusque, unresponsive, inattentive doctor who uses a rapid-fire questioning technique in an effort to get to the 'root of the problem'.

Individuals are more likely to comply with treatment if they understand the process of diagnosis and are involved in treatment decisions from the outset. This can only be facilitated through effective communication between doctor and patient. Gone are the days of shouting 'next patient please' into an

It is a **courtesy** to acknowledge your patient's attendance with a **warm greeting** and **handshake** intercom and making eye contact only with the strategically placed face of a watch!

It is a courtesy to acknowledge your patient's attendance with a warm greeting and handshake, offering physical help to negotiate furniture if required. It is clinically informative to observe the patient's mobility, and many practitioners now prefer to bypass the impersonal intercom and greet their patients in the waiting room. Scheduling for an appropriate duration of consultation is difficult but crucial. Table 1 outlines good

Table 1

Good practice during patient consultations

- Greet your patient warmly, confirming their name
- Observe their entrance and offer assistance if required
- Introduce yourself by name and job title
- Enquire about the reason for the patient's attendance today, remembering that they may not present with the complaint about which they are most concerned
- Maintain eye contact, be approachable and courteous
- Listen to, and avoid interrupting, the patient
- Avoid bypassing the patient, for example a child or the hard of hearing, by dealing only with the carer
- Avoid appearing rushed
- Select an appropriate approach, for example a doctor-led consultation (using more closed questions) for a patient with physical ill-health and a patient-led consultation (more open questions) where problems are predominantly psychosocial
- Provide a clear explanation of symptoms, diagnosis and treatment tailored to the patient's likely level of comprehension
- Involve the patient in decisions
- Acknowledge the rights to further opinions, confidentiality, privacy and dignity
- Offer additional support (e.g. from colleagues and documents)
- Close by summarizing and agree an agenda for follow-up

Table 2

Doctors' fears when giving bad news

- A lack of training, skills and experience
- Of being blamed for the diagnosis
- Of producing an adverse emotional reaction in a patient
- Of expressing their own emotions
- Of not knowing all the answers
- Personal fear of illness and death

practice during a patient consultation, which is both humane and clinically essential.

Breaking bad news and communicating with the dying are particularly stressful for doctor and patient, and warrant special consideration.

Breaking bad news

Breaking bad news is a particularly emotive area and one that demands particular skills. Bad news is information that a patient will perceive as being likely to change their own future dramatically, and picking up on a doctor's own anxieties and fears (Table 2) can make initiating the conversation difficult.

These fears should be recognized, as should the risk that the doctor may unconsciously assume 'responsibility' for the disease. Such an assumption of responsibility must be avoided as it can lead to a desire to shield and protect the patient. In turn, this can result in reduced comprehension and the doctor becoming a target for blame, making continued conversation with the patient increasingly difficult.

It is essential to control these emotions wherever possible, through awareness. At the same time, it must be appreciated that patients gain great benefit from well-expressed sympathy.

The doctor's tasks are to move the patient's attention gradually towards the reality of receiving news that is far less favourable than they might have hoped, to ensure comprehension and to give realistic hope (Table 3).

Table 3

Good practice when giving patients bad news

- Arrange a prompt consultation and encourage your patient to invite a relative or friend
- Ensure all essential clinical information is available and check the key facts, particularly proof of diagnosis
- Clarify the patient's existing level of knowledge
- Attempt to gauge how much the patient wants to know during the initial interaction and from previous assessment
- Do not be abrupt; give a warning shot – for example, state that the results may not be as good as was hoped
- Give the basic information, repeating important points and adding further information gradually
- Check repeatedly for understanding, and allow time for questions
- Empathize
- Encourage expression of feelings
- Offer help by identifying areas of major worry that can be prioritized and broken down into smaller items of concern
- Identify a plan of management and a broad time frame, giving hope in a realistic way
- Be there to support the patient in any way required
- Emphasize quality of life issues
- Summarize and offer written information
- Be flexible in arranging follow-up and offer to involve the partner or spouse

Communicating with dying patients

Palliative medicine is an expanding area of specialist practice requiring specific skills and training. It encompasses personal and professional, ethical, spiritual, cultural and teamwork issues. Effective communication with the dying patient can be facilitated by considering some key points, which can only be summarized here (Table 4).

Effective communication

Table 4

Communicating with dying patients

- Allow adequate time at each consultation
- Develop the confidence to deal with difficult questions
- Develop the skill of listening – accept that it is not possible to have a solution to every problem
- Use appropriate language and be prepared to repeat yourself
- Try to assess, without bias, what the patient really wants to know, rather than making assumptions about what the patient should know
- Give a strong message that you are still offering treatment to alleviate symptoms and concerns
- Explore anxieties – help to voice common ones, such as fear of pain, incontinence and dependence, and offer reassurance and advice
- Avoid giving a definite time span, but recognize the rate of deterioration and give advice based on this
- Be aware of your own inadequacies and be prepared to seek advice

It is essential to ensure that the relationship with the patient is based on honesty and openness. The doctor must try to overcome his or her own inadequacies and put aside any feelings of failure. Tactics to keep the patient at a safe emotional distance should be eschewed. Always attempt to put the patient's concerns first, ensuring full coverage of one topic before proceeding to the next set of problems. Offer frequent help and advice rather than leaving it to the patient to ask – they are likely to do so less frequently than needed. Determine whether help is required when communicating with loved ones. Give the reassurance of a fail-safe contact number.

> The **relationship** with the **patient** must be based on **honesty** and **openness**

Communicating with colleagues and managers

Practice colleagues

Good teamwork depends on unhindered and clear lines of communication between all team members. Colleagues in practice are a valuable resource for advice, and are often business partners and friends. Mutual respect is a cornerstone of a successful practice, enabling you to capitalize on the range of talents on offer. Regular practice meetings that allow contributions from all parties are essential.

In relation to clinical colleagues, it is common for everyone to feel as though they are doing the lion's share of the work. You should be generous with your help and time rather than trying to ensure that you do no more work than colleagues.

Colleagues in hospital practice

While it is important to recognize the benefit of advice from specialists, be confident rather than apologetic and uncertain when liaising with hospital colleagues. You have deemed the referral to be necessary and it will be you who resumes the care of your patient upon discharge. Recognize that you have skills that differ from and complement those of hospital specialists, and be aware that they also are working under pressure. Being aggressive and unreasonably demanding is unnecessary and counterproductive.

You have valuable first-hand knowledge of your patient, their history, treatments, behaviour, and family and socioeconomic status. Good clinical practice demands that all relevant information, including your own assessment of the situation, is relayed to the hospital team, preferably in writing. However, discussion of a clinical problem is often welcomed by hospital specialists and may serve to expedite or avoid the need for a referral.

Managers

A general practice is a complex organization, and the appointment of a suitably qualified manager makes excellent sense. Continuous involvement by clinicians in the minutiae of practice management does not.

A good manager relieves the partners of (and excels in) administrative issues. The doctor/manager relationship is thus likely to be one of equals in the practice team.

Practices in which one or more partners prefer to have more direct input into these duties will inevitably employ a manager who will be required to carry out decisions already made by the partners. The relationship will then be one of employer/employee, where the manager takes a more passive role. Whatever the structure, adhering to some key points (Table 5) is to be recommended.

Chairing small meetings and committees

Most of us will be required to chair a meeting at some time. You may well have experienced a meeting that should have been a very rapid and diplomatic way of reaching a consensus decision but which, instead, became a platform for the expression of long-winded and irrelevant discussion. The quality of the outcomes depends largely on the skills of the chairperson.

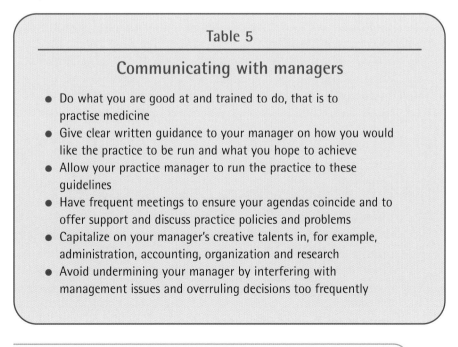

Table 5

Communicating with managers

- Do what you are good at and trained to do, that is to practise medicine
- Give clear written guidance to your manager on how you would like the practice to be run and what you hope to achieve
- Allow your practice manager to run the practice to these guidelines
- Have frequent meetings to ensure your agendas coincide and to offer support and discuss practice policies and problems
- Capitalize on your manager's creative talents in, for example, administration, accounting, organization and research
- Avoid undermining your manager by interfering with management issues and overruling decisions too frequently

Table 6

Chairing a meeting

- In advance, ensure the timely distribution of the agenda and relevant papers
- Ensure the appropriateness of the members and limit to essential contributors where possible
- Be familiar with the agenda, relevant documents and minutes of previous meetings – prioritize agenda items
- Appoint a non-contributor to keep minutes
- Ensure all members are introduced if they are not already familiar
- Seek approval for the minutes from the previous meeting
- Ensure recommended action from the previous meeting has been taken
- Proceed through the agenda, referring to all circulated and tabled documents, summarizing each successive discussion
- Limit discussion to salient points – politely terminate overlong contributions
- Invite contributions from less forward members
- Ensure a conclusion is reached for every agenda item and clarify this – postponement to a subsequent meeting may be acceptable in relation to some items
- Ensure duties are delegated and decide on a timetable
- Keep the whole meeting within its allocated time span
- Agree a date for the next meeting
- After the meeting, check the minutes for accuracy prior to circulation

A successful chairperson is one who is knowledgeable about the issues to be discussed and is sufficiently diplomatic and authoritative to encourage relevant contributions from all attendees while discouraging deviation. The chair should keep the meeting within its time allocation. Topics requiring prolonged discussion or further research should be postponed to another meeting or delegated as 'action points'. By following the guidance set out in Table 6, you may spare your colleagues from frustration and disappointment.

Making oral presentations

The aim is to deliver information clearly and concisely. Few can achieve this without practice and experience, but following some simple guidelines should help.

When preparing a presentation you should bear in mind that the concentration span of your audience is likely to be around 20 minutes. You may be able to extend this by varying the pace, the content and the type of images used, but you should ensure also that the main messages are delivered early and reiterated at the end. All but the most accomplished raconteurs choose to illustrate their discourse and the relative merits of various visual aids must be considered.

> The **concentration span** of your audience is likely to be around **20 minutes**

Overheads

Overheads are a simple and easy form of presentation. However, the incorporation of too much detail can be boring and difficult to follow. Avoid this by using large print with no more than six to eight lines of text per sheet. Avoid hand-written overheads at all costs!

Slides

Slides are a fairly simple and foolproof means of delivery, but take longer to prepare. They allow the introduction of images, which may help retain audience attention. Choose a clearly legible design, preferably pale text on a dark background. In general, don't try to cover more than one slide per minute of presentation time. Use no more than six lines of text per slide and do not employ complex tables. Avoid dual projection at all costs!

Computerized formats

Computerized formats (e.g. Microsoft PowerPoint) are a polished mode of presentation that is becoming the norm. In terms of content and layout, follow the guidance for slide presentations. Static and animated images can be used to help retain audience attention. You must ensure that there is equipment compatibility at the venue. Avoid multicoloured backgrounds (and moving ones, in particular) at all costs!

Preparation

Good preparation is essential if your presentation is to appear professional and, in turn, to be of value to the audience (key points are summarized in Table 7).

Delivery

Not all of us are gifted speakers, and many find the prospect of presenting to an audience positively daunting. There are, however, simple steps that you can take that will increase your confidence and enhance delivery; these are summarized in Table 8.

Making bids for resources

Successful bidding for resources to allow you to undertake projects/research in areas of particular interest can enhance job

---

Table 7

Good practice when preparing a presentation

- Prepare your presentation well in advance
- Keep it simple
- Include a clear introduction, preview of the content and concise conclusions
- Allow time to reiterate important details
- Rehearse your presentation before a friendly audience and listen to advice
- Rehearse the timing, allowing the designated period for discussion

---

Effective communication

Table 8
Advice on enhancing delivery

- Load and check through slides yourself
- Make yourself familiar with the podium equipment
- Remember, clarity is of fundamental importance
- Talk to the audience, not the screen nor the ceiling
- Do not speak down to your audience, nor try to confuse them
- Use a pointer for emphasis, but avoid lasering the audience
- Do not wander away (in particular, stay close to the microphone)
- Answer questions without aggression, and acknowledge the quality of the question if appropriate

satisfaction and improve the quality of service to your patients. All bids should include a work plan for resources and costings required for change. Some key points to address are shown in Table 9.

Information regarding making bids for resources in Wales and Northern Ireland can be obtained through the websites listed.

Bids to primary care trusts (PCTs) and groups (PCGs) (England)

PCTs are keen to smooth out inequalities of healthcare delivery by encouraging all practices to have basic provisions such as nursing care, a practice manager, and an accredited computer system. PCTs are also keen to take up bids for new GP initiatives by the use of non-recurrent money to finance pilot schemes, with a view to funding a wider uptake of successful projects.

> All **bids** should **include** the **resources** and the **costings** **required** for change

Should practices achieve targets for prescribing, bids may also be made for extra money from the prescribing incentive scheme.

Table 9

Items to include in bids for funding

Equipment
- Cost of initial outlay
- Provision for maintenance
- Planned usage
- Perceived benefit to practice and patient care

Staff employment
- Project outline – duration and benefits to practice and patients
- Staff grade and total cost
- Plans for further development

Research projects
- Project outline, feasibility and duration
- Resources required (e.g. stationery, equipment, cost of staff and training, transport, postage)
- Plans for dissemination of results
- Plans for shared costs

Items in the practice plan

At the beginning of each financial year, PCTs invite practices to include bids for items as part of their practice plan. These may include bids for additional staff, improvement of premises, equipment, health incentives, and courses.

Bids for slippage money

At the end of the financial year, practices may be invited to make bids for slippage money for short-term projects (slippage money is unspent money that cannot be carried over – it is non-recurrent money and thus is not to be used for ongoing employment). Possible items include improvement to computer systems, short-term projects (e.g. staffing costs for a named project), and one-off capital investments (e.g. installation of central heating).

Modernization funds

Bids can also be made to modernization funds held by PCTs. This money is intended to facilitate implementation of the new NHS plans. Bids could include plans to implement coronary heart disease policies or to modernize delivery of services to patients (for example, the development of outreach clinics).

Bids to local health care cooperatives (LHCC) (Scotland)

Bids for money originating from various sources, including the research development officer, should be made to the LHCC general manager. Bids are categorized and prioritized.

LHCC managers will invite practices to bid for available slippage money at the end of the financial year.

Bids to the national primary care collaborative

Groups of four to five practices can be financed to develop initiatives such as:
- improving the management of coronary heart disease
- making GP appointments accessible to patients
- improving referral systems to secondary care.

Bids for research and development funding

Research in primary care has, historically, been undertaken by enthusiastic individuals on an ad-hoc basis. However, increasingly GPs are making research grant applications themselves, or in conjunction with colleagues in secondary care, or university departments of general practice. Projects can vary from the design of a pharmaceutical trial to requests for protected time for research.

> **Projects** can **vary** from **trial design** to requests for **protected time** for research

Applications should be made to the relevant sub-committee of the Regional Offices (England) or Chief Scientist Office (Scotland) – website addresses are given on page 67. Research applications may also be made

Table 10

Making bids – some useful information

- Pre-prepared bids for projects can be kept on file for use at short notice
- Bids should be realistic – for some, rather than all, of the funds available
- It is useful to have one partner or manager who can search and apply for alternative sources of grants (and undertake the research)
- It is very important to ensure that the partnership agreement covers all items and equipment acquired, whatever the source of funding
- Health improvement managers may be a useful source of information regarding money available for bids
- Check appropriate websites (e.g. PCT, scot.nhs) to identify availability of untied money
- Make personal contact with individuals involved in allocation of resources (to help identify ongoing initiatives)

to Government bodies, Research Councils, charities or local endowment funds. General research databases (e.g. RDinfo) offer scope for further applications. Educational and financial support is also available for GPs who are just starting to develop their research careers from the Regional Offices or Chief Scientist Office, through Primary Care Research Networks.

Expertise in the development of research techniques may be developed by initial collaboration with university departments of general practice, which may be facilitated by the Trust's research and development officer.

Some useful information on bidding is summarized in Table 10.

Useful website addresses

National Health Service
http://www.nhs.uk

Department of Health, England
http://www.doh.gov.uk

Scottish Health
http://www.show.scot.nhs.uk/

NHS Wales
http://www.wales.nhs.uk/

HPSS, Northern Ireland
http://www.n-i.nhs.uk/

NHS Executive research funding digest (RDinfo)
http://www.rdinfo.org.uk

Chief Scientist Office
http://www.show.scot.nhs.uk/cso/

Further reading

Benson J, Britten N. Respecting the autonomy of cancer patents when talking with their families: qualitative analysis of semistructured interviews with patients. *BMJ* 1996;313:729–31.

Buckman R. *How To Break Bad News: A Guide For Healthcare Professionals.* London: Papermac, 1994.

Buckman R. *Talking to patients about cancer.* BMJ 1996;313:699–701.

Dickenson D, Johnson M. *Death, Dying and Bereavement.* London: Open University/Sage Publications, 1993.

Doyle D, Hanks G, McDonald N. *Oxford Textbook of Palliative Medicine* 2nd edn. Oxford: Oxford Medical Publications, 1999.

Fallowfield L. Giving sad and bad news. *Lancet* 1993;341:476–8.

Faulkner A, Argent J, Jones A *et al.* Improving the skills of doctors in giving distressing information. *Med Educ* 1995;29:303–7.

Flanagan, T. Doctor, do you have anything to say? *Medical Protection Society Casebook* 2000:15.

Ley P. *Communicating with Patients*. London: Chapman and Hall, 1988.

Lloyd M, Bor R. Communication Skills for Medicine. New York: Churchill Livingstone, 1996.

Neighbour R. *The inner consultation: how to develop an effective and intuitive consulting style*. Lancaster: MTP Press, 1987.

Pendleton D, Schofield T, Tate P *et al. The consultation: an approach to learning and teaching*. Oxford: Oxford University Press, 1984.

Silverman J, Kurtz S, Draper J. *Skills for Communicating with Patients*. Abingdon: Radcliffe Medical Press, 1988.

Effective communication

making **your mark** in **practice**

Dr Judy Gilley, Chief Executive,
Bedfordshire and Hertfordshire
Local Medical Committees

Choice and opportunity

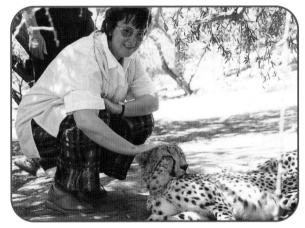

For today's aspiring GPs, opportunity and variety of career have never been greater. The days of working as a principal in the same practice for 30 years, with a 'flat career pathway' are numbered. You can indeed still opt for traditional practice as a self-employed principal with the security and pleasures of providing continuity of care for patients over a working lifetime. Alternatively, you may decide to change practices for variety of experience. Or you may choose to work in a salaried capacity, perhaps in a personal medical services (PMS) scheme with limited working hours and a short-term contract. A period of locum work can provide valuable insight into a variety of practices and help you decide what type of practice is right for you. Interest is growing in such 'portfolio careers'.

> For today's **GPs, opportunity** and **variety** of career have **never** been **greater**

Flexible working

For the increasing number of women achieving a vocational training certificate, the early years in practice may be the best time for starting a family. Part-time flexible working is possible in both conventional general medical services (GMS) and the PMS schemes. The popular doctors' retainer scheme aims to keep doctors with a domestic commitment in touch with medicine by financial support for practices employing them for up to four sessions a week. Local postgraduate deaneries oversee the scheme, which includes ongoing educational support for retainers.

Further training

Many GP registrars take Membership of the Royal College of General Practitioners (MRCGP) during their registrar year although this produces a demanding schedule. Increasingly, general practice offers possibilities for higher postgraduate training and qualifications, or a career combining clinical and academic general practice. More young doctors are opting to learn research methodology to enrich their clinical practice and to contribute to the research base that is so urgently needed in primary care.

> Many **learn** research methodology to **enrich** their clinical **practice**

Generalist versus specialist

The debate about whether GPs should be dedicated generalists or should also opt for 'specialisms' has intensified with the NHS Plan. Some GPs are opting for additional training for approval to perform traditional hospital-based services, such as surgery, endoscopy, and dermatology in the practice setting. The aim is to enhance patient access to services by GPs developing their 'special interest'.

Defining success

So the world really is your oyster as a young GP. The problem is how to define what you want from a diverse career, and to decide what

Making your mark in practice

constitutes success and satisfaction for you. It is likely that you will define success in different ways at different stages of your career.

Success from the patient's perspective

Success must be grounded in achieving the approval and trust of patients who want a GP who is kind, trustworthy, keeps confidence with them, and involves them in decision-making about treatment options. In other words, a doctor who is a good communicator, and keeps up to date with clinical practice. Today's GP also needs to demonstrate their quality of practice by recording outcomes and undertaking regular audits.

Success from local population initiatives

Traditionally, general practice focused on the individual patient, but today's GP needs an additional 'population focus.' This means setting up systems to detect 'at risk' patients in the practice population, and coding risk and disease categories to target patients with appropriate preventive measures and treatments.

The use of computers, opportunities for data collection and analysis, and for achieving national service framework targets are all hallmarks of our increasingly sophisticated ability to improve the health of populations. Demonstrating that you have made a difference can be very satisfying professionally.

Success in team working

Success has also to be defined in terms of the ability of the GP to organize decent facilities for patients within limited financial resources, including the creation of multiprofessional teams. GPs need to be confident team players, and often team leaders. You may have your vision of the future, and find success in motivating your team to share and achieve that vision.

Success as perceived by colleagues

Success may mean winning the approval and respect of your colleagues, not only within the practice, but also in the wider medical community. You can make significant contributions to patient care by undertaking a bewildering range of activities outside your practice. These may include active participation in the local Royal College of General Practitioners (RCGP) faculty, or working as a GP member of the local primary care organization, for example as an executive member of your primary care trust. Being elected to represent GPs on your Local Medical Committee (LMC) is an indication that you are seen as understanding general practice, and trusted to act altruistically in the best interests of general practice and of GP colleagues. These opportunities to engage with new people and new ideas are an antidote to professional isolation and stagnation.

Success as a trainer

One-quarter of practices are training practices. In order to train GP registrars, you and your practice must be approved periodically. The support of your partners is, therefore, essential. Training offers enormous rewards, including better understanding of your own learning style (activist, reflector, theorist, or pragmatist?) and the chance to help colleagues achieve their career aspirations.

> **Training** offers **enormous rewards**

Success in terms of earning capacity

General practice offers the flexibility of non-NHS work to supplement NHS earnings, and a greater percentage of GPs' income is now derived from non-GMS sources. GPs' earnings vary considerably both from NHS and non-NHS work. It is essential that you take out adequate income protection against incapacity.

GMS GPs

GMS GPs should see the practice accounts and take expert accountancy advice before joining a practice. The Doctors and Dentists Review Body determines the average pay for GMS GPs, but you must be confident of your fair share of the practice profits as reflected in your partnership agreement. The General Practitioners Committee of the BMA negotiates the national contract for GPs.

PMS GPs

If you join a PMS scheme you are entering a local agreement and will need expert advice on the financial rewards and terms of service implications of your contract with your primary care trust (PCT).

Salaried GPs

If you work in a salaried capacity, either within GMS or PMS, you need expert advice (from the BMA, your LMC, legal or accountancy advisor) as to the terms and conditions of service and pay in your contract.

Finding your focus

Talking to colleagues and your trainer may help you to understand where your future lies. Expert advice may be available from your local postgraduate deanery, The Medical Women's Federation, your RCGP faculty, or your LMC. A university department of primary care can be a good starting point for discussing a career in academic general practice.

> You may **feel inspired** to shape healthcare policy **via** a career in **medical politics**

You may wish to immerse yourself in clinical work, undertake further training or degrees, or develop your research skills. You may be interested in becoming a trainer. If you are attracted to management you may want to work for your PCT and consider a management qualification. You may feel inspired to shape healthcare policy via a career in medical politics. Membership of your LMC may lead to regional and national representative bodies, such as the General Practitioners' Committee of the BMA.

Taking control

Home/work balance

It is possible to adjust your workload at different life stages by changing your contractual arrangements. At all times, achieving an acceptable home/work balance is crucial. Younger GPs correctly reject the excessive working hours of their predecessors. GPs are sensitive to the consequences of too little quality time for children. Time for relaxation with family and friends, and for interests outside medicine are all absolutely essential. Variety can reduce stress and burnout.

Your skills are in demand

The shortage of GPs means that working arrangements are becoming more sensitive to doctors' needs. There are more opportunities for flexible working. Be prepared to search them out.

Practice/external work balance

Getting the right balance between practice responsibilities and outside medical activities is also crucial. If you spend too much time (particularly unremunerated) outside the practice, you may generate tensions and disharmony. Transparency with your partners and team is essential, and seeking agreement prior to undertaking outside activities is crucial (and usually set out in the partnership agreement). Your absence means others have to pick up your work, and the practice needs to be compensated financially.

> The **right balance** between practice responsibilities and outside activities **is crucial**

Building clinical expertise

Lifelong learning

Today's GP will need to plan for a lifetime of learning to keep pace with the complexity of modern medicine and for revalidation purposes. Rigid systems of lecture-based learning are slowly being transformed into multiple learning opportunities. GPs and other members of practice teams are being encouraged to produce personal development plans. Distance learning, mentoring arrangements, and 'practice learning days' when all local practices close for a shared study afternoon, are all happening.

Opportunities for prolonged study leave are still rare and costly for self-employed GPs. Some practices include sabbaticals in partnership agreements, but these are usually self-financing.

Appraisal and revalidation

The moves towards annual appraisal of doctors and revalidation are already driving a cultural change involving routine demonstration of satisfactory practice. Revalidation builds on the foundation of the GMC's standards set out in *Good Medical Practice*. It is likely to be based on the periodic review of a folder of evidence collected by each GP describing 'what the doctor does and how well the doctor does it'.

> Moves towards appraisal and revalidation are already driving a cultural change

Special interests

More GPs may choose to train for approval for 'specialisms' and to undertake patient referrals from other GPs. It will be crucial that the distinct generalist skills of GPs are not sacrificed to multiple mini-specialisms. Many local development schemes exist for enhancing traditional work, for example by more organized chronic-disease management. These schemes can be highly satisfying.

Managing demand

Time management techniques

Time management techniques will be your survival skill, and some good courses are available. Effective management of paperwork and telephone time, appropriate delegation and saying 'no' all help, as does a good practice manager. Successive governments have sought to reduce bureaucracy, but it has the habit of reinventing itself.

Communication skills and effective working techniques

The move to electronic records demands computer-based skills, and there are many good courses organized by both computer suppliers and the local NHS. However, well-structured 'face-to-face' meetings will remain essential for healthy team working. Every meeting needs a clear purpose, agreed agenda, and cut-off time. Decisions and action points must be recorded and acted upon. Professional time is a scarce commodity.

Well-structured 'face-to-face' meetings remain essential for healthy team working

Good communications with secondary care are also crucial for success, by clear referral letters or use of agreed local direct-booking protocols. Unfortunately, there seems to be less face-to-face communication between GPs and consultant colleagues. It may be that e-mail will reverse this trend.

Learning from criticism

Patients are finding their voices, and are more likely to produce criticisms and to complain. Defensive reactions are not helpful to either party; no doctor is infallible and we can all learn from complaints. Many complaints derive from system failures, and you need to try to improve your practice systems if this is what your investigation reveals.

You need to be confident that you understand the NHS complaints arrangements and have a good in-house system (most complaints are resolved 'in house'). Never fire off a letter in hasty response to a complaint, always sleep on it and ask for the views of your colleagues before responding. Expert advice and support is available from your defence organization and your LMC.

Be prepared to look openly at criticisms, to be honest and open in your responses, and change your practice if necessary. These steps can strengthen your working relationships with your patients and your own confidence in your quality of practice.

Further reading

Bache J, Thomson A. Developing a secondary career. Career Focus. *BMJ Classified*, 17 February 2001: 2–3.

Baker M, Pringle M. Is there a future for independent contractor status in UK general practice? London: Royal College of General Practitioners Publications, 2000.

Fugelli P. Professional trust in general practice. The James MacKenzie Lecture 2000. London: Royal College of General Practitioners Publications, 2000.

The GP Retainer Scheme. Guidance from the General Practitioners Committee. London: British Medical Association, April 2000.

Handysides S. Returning to general practice. Career Focus. *BMJ Classified*, 20 January 2001: 2–3.

Harrison J, Innes R, Van Zwannenberg T. *The New GP: Changing Roles and the Modern NHS.* Abingdon: Radcliffe Medical Press, 2001.

Penchelon D, Mien Koh Y. Leadership and motivation. Career Focus. *BMJ Classified*, 29 July 2000: 2–3.

Willis J. *Friends in Low Places.* Abingdon: Radcliffe Medical Press, 2001.

managing a practice

Mr David Grantham,
Industrial Relations Officer of the BMA

Proper practice management is essential to being a successful GP. It is, however, an area most experts would agree is overlooked in GP training. What are the most important elements that need to be considered and how do you avoid the common pitfalls? Key problem areas are staffing, premises and information technology (IT), and whatever support GPs may have from a practice manager, the successful GP needs to be conversant with these issues.

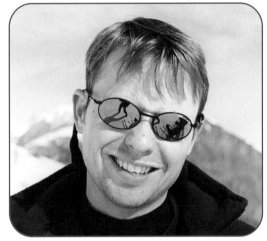

Key problem areas in managing a practice are **staffing, premises** and **IT**

Managing staff

All but the smallest of practices will now commonly employ a practice manager who will take the lead in managing staff. Nevertheless in GP partnerships (still the most common practice arrangement), it is the partners who are ultimately responsible for the health, safety and welfare of their employees. It is vital that all the partners have an understanding of these responsibilities as employees are better protected than ever before in terms of the benefits they enjoy and their ability to enforce those rights against employers (Table 1).

Table 1

Principal employment rights

Individual employment right	Qualifying service necessary
• To be given a minimum period of notice – based on length of service – of termination of employment	4 weeks
• To be given written particulars of terms of employment	8 weeks
• To receive equal pay with a member of the opposite sex doing similar work	Applies immediately
• Not to be discriminated against on the grounds of marriage or sex	Any stage, from advertising of job onwards
• Not to be discriminated against on the grounds of colour, race, nationality, or ethnic or national origin	Any stage, from advertising of job onwards
• Not to be discriminated against on grounds of disability	Any stage, from advertising of job (applies if 16 or more employees)
• Not to be unfairly dismissed	1 year†
• Not to be dismissed on pregnancy or childbirth grounds	Applies immediately
• To take 18 weeks' maternity leave*	Applies immediately
• To return to work up to 29 weeks after week in which childbirth occurs	1 year
• To have unpaid time off for public duties	Applies immediately

Table 1 (continued)

Principal employment rights

Individual employment right	Qualifying service necessary
• To have time off – with pay – to seek alternative work or to arrange training if made redundant	2 years
• To receive statutory minimum paid holidays (4 weeks)	Applies immediately
• To receive an itemized pay statement	Applies immediately
• To receive on request a written statement of the reason for dismissal	1 year (immediately and automatically if for pregnancy reasons)
• To have paid time off for antenatal care	Applies immediately
• To be paid at least the national minimum wage	Applies immediately
• To have unpaid time off for paternity and special domestic leave*	Applies immediately

*Changes are proposed to increase maternity leave to 26 weeks from April 2003, and to introduce 2 weeks' paid paternity leave.
†If dismissal is for certain inadmissible reasons – that is, for reasons of trade union membership or activities, maternity or childbirth, or discrimination – there is no length of service qualification.

Keeping up to date with changes in employment legislation is a difficult task, but employers who don't do so run the risk of compensation claims in employment tribunals running into many thousands of pounds. The employment tribunal is the judicial forum in which employees can seek redress for breaches of their employment rights or contracts of employment.

However, in line with the growth in employment legislation, there has also been an expansion in the range of advice and guidance available to small employers (including practices). Much of this is accessible via the worldwide web and through advisory organizations. Some good sources of up-to-date guidance and websites are listed on page 91.

Recommendation

Make sure someone in the practice is charged with maintaining a watching brief over employment issues and, therefore, that the practice remains up to date.

Recruitment, selection and staff contracts

Proper procedures for the recruitment and selection of staff are vital. Before seeking to advertise, a proper job description should be prepared and, if possible, a person specification setting out desirable qualifications, experience and characteristics. This will help the partners make their decision after the interviews. There must be no discrimination on grounds of race or sex when making recruitment decisions. That means that decisions to appoint must be based on an objective assessment of an individual's abilities regardless of their sex or race. Partners must be prepared to justify decisions in the face of any challenge.

Once appointed, staff must receive a written statement of the main terms of their employment within 8 weeks of starting work. The items the statement must deal with are listed in Table 2. Additional items recommended for inclusion are given in Table 3.

The reason all staff should have written contracts of employment is to avoid disputes about the terms on which the employee has been engaged.

Recommendation

In the first instance, staff should be engaged for a probationary period, usually 3–6 months, during which time satisfactory performance can be confirmed. Employment should also be offered subject to satisfactory

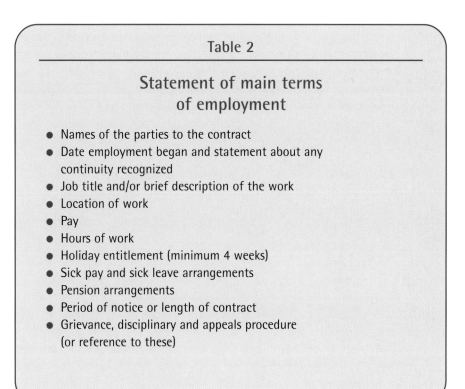

Table 2

Statement of main terms of employment

- Names of the parties to the contract
- Date employment began and statement about any continuity recognized
- Job title and/or brief description of the work
- Location of work
- Pay
- Hours of work
- Holiday entitlement (minimum 4 weeks)
- Sick pay and sick leave arrangements
- Pension arrangements
- Period of notice or length of contract
- Grievance, disciplinary and appeals procedure (or reference to these)

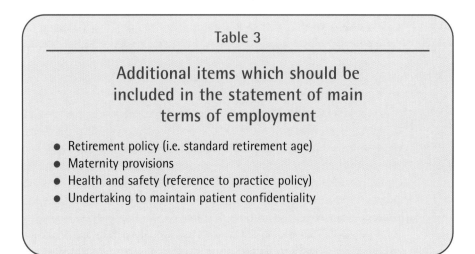

Table 3

Additional items which should be included in the statement of main terms of employment

- Retirement policy (i.e. standard retirement age)
- Maternity provisions
- Health and safety (reference to practice policy)
- Undertaking to maintain patient confidentiality

references. These can be taken up prior to or during the probationary period. From then on, regular appraisal of staff and review of any contracts that are superseded are strongly advised (e.g. as new tasks are taken on or hours changed). A word of caution, however, it is important to note that changes to contracts of employment should not be imposed unilaterally, but only following consultation with the staff affected.

Disciplinary and grievance procedures

All employers are now required to let employees know of their disciplinary and grievance procedures or rules. These must be notified to new employees within 8 weeks of appointment.

The disciplinary procedure sets out the steps that will be taken against employees who are failing to perform their duties satisfactorily or are otherwise in breach of the contract of employment, for example by consistently arriving late. It should also explain that gross misconduct (e.g. theft or breach of patient confidentiality) might lead to summary dismissal (instant dismissal without notice) once a formal disciplinary hearing has been held.

> New employees must be **notified** of disciplinary and grievance **procedures**

Failure to follow a fair disciplinary procedure in dismissing an employee is very likely to give an employee grounds for complaint to an employment tribunal. The fair procedure that should be followed is set out in the Advisory Conciliation and Arbitration Service (ACAS) code (see 'Further information', page 91).

Employees have the right to be accompanied by a fellow employee or union representative at disciplinary and grievance hearings if the request is reasonable (i.e. the representative can attend within a reasonable period and is not someone who is involved with the matter under discussion). If the representative cannot attend on the date proposed, the hearing must be postponed for up to 5 working days to allow alternative representation.

A grievance procedure is the steps an employee may take to have concerns or disputes with their employer considered. Usually this will involve first raising the matter with the immediate line manager and, if matters cannot be resolved, consideration of the issues by a higher authority, usually the partners. It is necessary to have such procedures written down so employees are aware how they may pursue complaints or concerns.

Recommendation

ACAS produces an excellent handbook on disciplinary procedures for employers, obtainable from local ACAS enquiry points or at www.acas.org.uk. The ACAS guide sets the standard against which employers' procedures are judged whenever challenged in the employment tribunal by an employee they have dismissed. Make sure you have an up-to-date copy.

Relationships with unions

Many staff are members of a trade union. In larger workplaces (more than 21 employees), unions may request recognition for the purposes of collective bargaining (negotiating on terms and conditions on behalf of all employees). If recognition is refused, a statutory procedure may be followed to force the employer to grant recognition. This is a complicated process involving a ballot of the workers. If a majority of those voting in a ballot in which 40% of the workforce have participated vote for recognition, the employer must grant recognition.

> There are **statutory provisions** governing **union recognition**

Not all practices will have more than 21 employees, but those that do should be mindful of the statutory provisions governing union recognition. Indeed, if a request for recognition is received, the best advice is to secure voluntary agreement of the terms on which the union making the request will be recognized to avoid the complicated statutory process.

For employers with fewer than 21 employees, there is no requirement to recognize trade unions for the purposes of collective bargaining. The only contact such practices are likely to have is with local union representatives when employees exercise their right to be accompanied at disciplinary and grievance hearings.

Problems with premises

Premises can often cause problems in general practice. Usually the problems will relate to development (dealt with later), ownership, valuation and leases. Disputes can be costly, as the legal issues involved can be complex and specialist advice may be required. The best way of avoiding difficulties is to make sure that the ownership, valuation and lease arrangements are clearly written down in the form of proper agreements.

In most practices some, but perhaps not all, of the partners will own the premises and receive reimbursement from the health authority for the cost of providing these premises to the NHS. Where this is the case, the partnership agreement must specify the arrangements for transfer of ownership, including valuation, on the death or retirement of a partner. If there are non-property-owning partners, the terms on which they might continue to occupy the premises for a limited period on leaving the partnership ought also to be included. Note that, under the NHS Acts, transfers of property between outgoing and incoming GP partners must not involve any element of 'goodwill'. A 'sale of goodwill' is prohibited under the NHS Acts and may be found to have arisen if an incoming partner pays more than the current market value of the practice premises being transferred.

The other arrangement is the occupation of premises owned by a third party (NHS trust, private landlord or property developer). Here, the practice must have a proper lease agreement setting out the terms of their occupation of the premises and the respective responsibilities of leaseholder and lessee.

The **advice** of a **lawyer** is probably worthwhile when **buying premises**

Where joint ownership with a third party is contemplated, it is again vital that the terms of occupation are in the form of a written agreement with that third party.

Recommendation

Investment in practice premises (buying premises or taking a lease) is as serious a business as buying or leasing your home. This is one instance in which the advice of a lawyer is probably a worthwhile expense, even if only to satisfy you that there are no hidden pitfalls in the purchase or lease arrangement proposed.

Developing premises

The NHS Plan has set an ambitious plan for improving GP premises by 2004. Over £1 billion is promised to develop 500 primary care centres and improve 3000 existing GP premises. Some of this money will be distributed under new schemes in addition to the traditional mechanisms for funding GP premises under the cost and notional rent schemes, and through improvement grants.

Central to the government's plan is the involvement of the private sector in developing new premises often in multi-occupancy units which, in addition to space for GP services, might provide room for other retail and office leaseholders, thereby spreading the costs of development. The key headache in such developments is the complexity generated by a larger range of stakeholders who each have an interest in how the development proceeds.

However, to encourage GPs to consider such arrangements and to discard premises no longer suited to the needs of modern practice, health authorities are able to make use of eight new flexible options (Table 4).

Recommendation

Investment in premises involves a risk and, in considering the development or improvement of premises, you must make a careful appraisal of the potential consequences of any investment you may make personally. In the mid-1990s, many GPs who had borrowed under the cost-rent scheme to invest in premises found that depressed property prices meant they did not receive the return they expected. However, the converse may also be true when property prices rise rapidly.

Table 4

New premises – flexible options for authorities

- Leasing premises directly to 'sub-let' them to GPs, when GPs are themselves reluctant to enter into long-term lease arrangements with the developer/owner of premises
- Increasing rent reimbursement to more than that based on current market value
- Funding the re-conversion of owner occupied premises back to residential accommodation for sale
- Guaranteeing GPs a minimum price for the sale of their premises
- Entering into joint lease ventures with third parties
- Reconverting properties for social landlord purposes (e.g. residential accommodation above the practice premises)
- Offering reimbursement of the costs of leasing equipment in new leasehold premises
- Developing mobile service delivery units (i.e. funding transportable premises)

Information technology

IT investments within the wider NHS do not have an entirely happy history and the same is true in general practice. Nevertheless, careful IT investment is an essential part of running a successful practice by improving administration and record keeping, as well as providing a valuable tool for audit and research. Nowadays, Internet access also provides a wealth of sources of information.

Careful IT investment is an **essential** part of a **successful** practice

Practices can receive support from the health authority (through primary care groups and trusts) for the costs of expenditure on computer infrastructure, and staff reimbursement, for system operators/data-entry clerks. However, to receive such reimbursement the system purchased must be one accredited by the Department of Health.

Since 2000, it has been legitimate to hold patient records on practice computer systems in place of paper records, provided the system:

- is secure
- can demonstrate an audit trail (that is, all amendments to data can be tracked by date and time)
- can provide a satisfactory printed record for transfer to the patient's next GP or health authority (practices should obtain a copy of the *Good Practice Guidelines for GP Electronic Patient Records* prepared by the Royal College of General Practitioners and General Practitioners' Committee, BMA).

Practices holding patient-identifiable data must be registered with the Data Protection Registrar and have to comply with data protection legislation. This governs patients' rights of access, and the rules regarding disclosure and use of information held. The basic rule is that patient confidentiality must be rigorously protected. Practice staff must adhere to this. Practices are also well advised to have a clear policy on Internet usage by staff.

Recommendation

There are many computer systems on the market. Practices are best advised to discuss future development of systems with the health authority, primary care group or trust, as many now have policies of only reimbursing systems that meet local requirements regarding compatibility between practices.

Maximizing your income

The obvious first step in maximizing income is to ensure that the practice is receiving the correct reimbursements from the health authority or trust. That means checking that all the claims that could have been made have been submitted and that these have been paid. For those under a personal medical services (PMS) contract, there are no such claims as a fixed sum is usually paid each month.

The second step is to make sure that all partners are aware of the limited range of circumstances in which additional charges can be made from patients or third parties for services provided. An example is travel vaccinations for which no fee is payable by the health authority. The circumstances in which GPs may charge NHS patients are set out in paragraph 38 of the terms of service.

The third step is to look to new sources of income by either providing new NHS services under separate contract with the health authority (under general medical services local development schemes or as part of a PMS+ contract) or undertaking work for a local hospital or privately. Local medical committees (LMCs) and the health authority or trust should be able to advise of any such schemes in operation (for example for care of asylum seekers).

There are **plenty** of **opportunities** for **boosting earnings**

Finally, opportunities in medical writing, medical advisory/assessment services, occupational health, sports medicine, education and training are there to be exploited. If you have the relevant skills and the time available, there are plenty of opportunities for boosting non-NHS earnings.

Recommendation

Be imaginative in considering the options for work outside the NHS. Not only can such activities be rewarding, financially, they can help provide variety in your practice and a relief from the routine day-to-day surgery.

Further information

Advisory Conciliation and Arbitration Service (ACAS)

Employing People – a Handbook for Small Firms
Discipline at Work
Employment Handbook
Publications: 01455 852225
Website: www.acas.org.uk

Department of Trade and Industry

Guide to the Working Time Regulations
Maternity Rights: A Guide for Employers and Employees
Parental Leave: A Guide for Employers and Employees
Fair and Unfair Dismissal: A Guide for Employers
Individual Rights of Employees: A Guide for Employers and Employees
Contracts of Employment
Publications: 0870 1502 500
Website: www.dti.gov.uk/er

DTI Small business service

Disability Discrimination in Employment URN 00/960
Dismissal: Fair or Unfair? URN 00/952
Itemised Pay Statements URN 00/953
Maternity Rights URN 00/954
National Minimum Wage URN 00/951
Part-time Workers URN 00/1132
Racial Discrimination in Employment URN 00/959
Redundancy URN 00/956
Sex Discrimination and Equal Pay URN 00/958
Publications: 0870 1502 500
Website: www.businessadviceonline.org

BMA

Model Contracts of Employment for Salaried GPs, Assistants, Retainees and GP Registrars
Model Contract and Staff Handbook for GP (Non-medical) Staff
Guidelines for Good Practice in the Recruitment and Selection of Doctors
Health and Safety at Work – Guidance for GPs (BMA General Practitioners' Committee)
Publications: members only through local offices
Website: www.bma.org.uk

clinical governance and self-regulation

Sir Donald Irvine CBE,
President of the General Medical Council

In the UK, almost everyone is registered with a family doctor. Patients expect their doctors to put their interests first, to be knowledgeable and skilful, empathetic, good communicators, and honest and truthful.

At the practice, patients expect good access to care and an appropriate range of medical and health services. Their trust in their doctor and the practice team stems partly from their personal experience and partly from their belief that the NHS, the medical profession and the practice have systems in place that ensure good care.

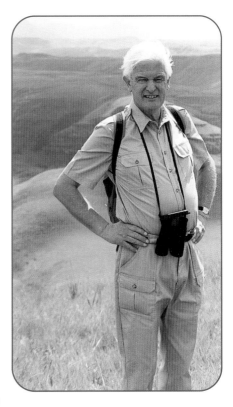

The regulatory framework

Medical practice is regulated by the profession itself, by contract and by the legal system. The General Medical Council (GMC) licenses doctors to practise. It derives its authority from the Medical Act, the purpose of which is to make sure that only doctors who are honest and reliable care for the public in this country.

Professional self-regulation

Professional self-regulation is a privilege not a right. There are three main reasons why professional self-regulation should give the public the best results provided that it works well. First, the scientific and technical complexity of medicine is such that it needs to be regulated by people who understand it. Secondly, patients are critically dependent on the ability and conscientiousness of their doctor to make the right decisions for them. Doctors are most likely to perform well when they are committed to a code of professional values and standards that constitute the profession's collective conscience. And thirdly, doctors are best placed to protect patients from colleagues whose practice gives cause for concern.

> Professional **self-regulation** is a **privilege not** a **right**

Professional self-regulation is changing in all professions. In medicine, this is partly because the public wants a greater say, particularly on those aspects of practice where the patient's perceptions of quality are paramount. The likely outcome will be a system that will continue to be professionally led, but which will represent more of an equal partnership between the medical profession and the public.

GMC

The GMC works by maintaining a register of those it considers to be competent to practise. To give effect to this in today's context, it is introducing far-reaching changes (Table 1).

The Royal College of General Practitioners (RCGP)

The Royal College of General Practitioners (RCGP), working alongside the GMC, sets specific professional standards for general practice and certifies the achievement of these by individual doctors through its Membership examination and Fellowship by assessment.

The Joint Committee on Postgraduate Training for General Practice

The Joint Committee on Postgraduate Training for General Practice supervises the training of new GPs.

<table>
Table 1

Changes being introduced by the General Medical Council

- A statement of the duties and responsibilities of doctors, as set out in *Good Medical Practice*, which codifies what the public and the medical profession agree should be expected of a doctor
- The explicit linkage of these professional standards with GMC registration, so that individual doctors can be held properly to account for their competence, performance and conduct through the regular checks on their practice needed to revalidate their registration every 5 years
- Changes to medical education to ensure, at all stages, that the system produces doctors with the attributes and qualities required for GMC registration
- New arrangements for dealing promptly and fairly with concerns about doctors whose conduct, performance or health may bring their registration into question
</table>

The local medical committees

The local medical committees provide local professional networks that are often invoked to help deal with doctors whose practice is questionable.

Clinical governance

Clinical governance is defined as "a framework through which NHS organizations are accountable for continuously improving the quality of their services and safeguarding high standards of care by creating an environment in which excellence in clinical care will flourish" (Secretary of State for Health, 1998). In practical terms, clinical governance is, therefore, the application of the principles of good management practice to the clinical process.

Clinical governance forms part of a wider framework for medical regulation introduced by the Government. The Government's quality agenda (Secretary of State for Health, 2001) is predicated on the principles of continuous quality improvement (CQI) and quality assurance. In its NHS modernization programme, it has institutionalized the various elements of CQI and quality assurance. National clinical guidelines in England are set by the National Institute for Clinical Excellence (NICE). External performance review is carried out by the Commission for Health Improvement in England and the Clinical Standards Board in Scotland. The National Service Frameworks provide a management instrument for seeking optimum results in priority clinical areas. The proposed system for recording clinical incidents is described in *An Organisation with a Memory*. And the new National Clinical Assessment Authority will make a preliminary assessment of GPs who may be underperforming, with the object of helping to restore them to fully effective practice.

These measures, and the profession's own regulatory framework, only make sense if they are seen as a mosaic in which each part has a distinct, well-defined function and the whole is well coordinated.

Impact on everyday professional life

While being aware of the regulatory system, most GPs just want to get on with their own practice. It may be helpful to summarize those elements that will be important to every doctor.

Professional standards and values

Every GP must be familiar with the duties and responsibilities of a doctor set out by the GMC in the booklet *Good Medical Practice*. These duties have been translated recently by the RCGP and the General Practitioners' Committee specifically into the context of general practice, in the booklet *Good Medical Practice for General Practitioners*.

GPs are expected to practise in accordance with these principles – they are not optional extras.

Ensuring good medical practice – revalidation

Both the Government and the GMC are introducing complementary arrangements to make sure that individual doctors can demonstrate that they are keeping up-to-date and providing a good standard of practice and care.

There are two ways of achieving this. Each year, GPs will be asked to undergo an appraisal of their work by their peers. This will be done locally under arrangements established by the primary care group or trust. The appraisal, against the template of *Good Medical Practice*, should draw on information about the doctor's practice that has been generated largely within the practice through the processes of clinical governance.

Appraisal, to be effective, should be a formative, supportive process. Of course it is a review of performance. But it should be more than that. It should be used as a positive aid to the doctor's professional development. And it should provide the doctor with the opportunity of setting out constraints in the practice environment – over which he or she may have little or no control – which are felt to be factors limiting good performance.

> Every **5 years,** GPs will be asked to **submit evidence** for **revalidation**

Revalidation is at 5-yearly intervals. GPs will be asked to submit to the GMC evidence, based on the yearly appraisals, that describes their performance in practice. The evidence will be assessed by a local panel of professional colleagues and members of the public appointed by the GMC.

GPs who practise conscientiously and keep themselves up-to-date should have nothing to fear from these processes. On the contrary, 30 years' experience with a similar process for appointing and reappointing trainers and teaching practices has shown how professionally motivating regular peer review can be. If problems with practice arise, they should be spotted early and the doctor given the chance and the opportunity to put things right. So all doctors who approach these local reviews of practice conscientiously should look forward with confidence to being revalidated. It is those who have not taken their professional responsibilities as seriously as they ought to, who may find their registration in question.

Clinical governance – the practice team

Clinical governance is very much a team-based business. For the patient, the quality of care depends partly on the knowledge, skills and attitudes of individual practitioners. But it depends equally on the way in which the practice as a whole delivers care.

Modern practice management is simply clinical governance under a more familiar name. The objective is straightforward. Practices need to be clear about the range of services they offer and their objectives for care. They need to show whether the practice as a whole, and its individual members, are achieving these objectives. This implies good records, good data, and good internal systems of clinical audit, risk management and so on. They need to be sure that each member of the practice has the time and avails themselves of the opportunities to further their own training and professional development. When problems or complaints arise, the practice needs to be able to deal with these promptly and effectively to minimize the risk to patients and damage to the individual team member.

These ideas are not new. A growing number of practices already work this way. What is becoming much more explicit is the idea of collective responsibility within a practice team for the quality of care. Practices that share such responsibility have found the benefit, in terms of feeling more in control of their own lives and destinies, important for morale.

In 1998, the GMC set out its basic requirements for clinical governance in clinical teams in the booklet *Maintaining Good Medical Practice*.

In conclusion

Changes in the regulatory framework will have a **direct** impact on **every GP**

Changes taking place in the regulatory framework of medicine today will have a direct impact on the lives of every GP. These are changes that the medical profession, the public and government think are necessary to make sure that practice in the future is as safe and effective as possible. They are becoming an integral part of modern practice for all doctors.

Further reading

General Medical Council. *Good Medical Practice.* 2nd edn. London: GMC, 1998.

General Medical Council. *Maintaining Good Medical Practice.* London: GMC, 1998.

Harrison, J, Van Zwanenberg, T. *Clinical Governance in Primary Care.* Oxford: Radcliffe Medical Press, 1999.

Irvine D, Irvine S. *The Practice of Quality.* Oxford: Radcliffe Medical Press, 1999.

Irvine DH. The performance of doctors. I: Professionalism and self regulation in a changing world. *BMJ* 1997;314:1540–2.

Royal College of General Practitioners. *Good Medical Practice for General Practitioners.* London: RCGP, 2000.

Secretary of State for Health. *A First Class Service: Quality in the New NHS.* London: Department of Health, 1998.

Secretary of State for Health. *An Organisation with a Memory.* London: Department of Health, 2000.

Secretary of State for Health. *Assuring the Quality of Practice: Implementing Supporting Doctors Protecting Patients.* London: Department of Health, 2001.

finance

Mrs Valerie Martin,
PKF Chartered Accountants

The greatest surprise to many doctors on starting their professional lives as a GP principal is the concept of being self-employed. Throughout your time as a junior doctor and GP registrar you will have been an employee of the NHS and taxed under the PAYE system, so it has not been necessary to give any consideration to understanding how businesses are run and how the tax system works. Now, as a GP, you will be self-employed and need some

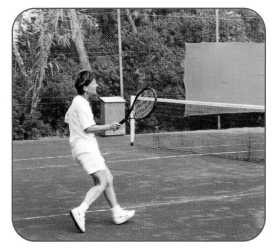

knowledge of the business side of general practice, and to understand a set of accounts and how the UK tax system works.

Before committing yourself to joining any partnership you need to ensure that you have the same work ethos as your prospective partners. If you are keen to work very hard and make as much money as possible from the practice, you don't want to find that your partners are more interested in lifestyle decisions and using locums to ease their workload. Conversely, if you would like to earn a little less and have some spare

> Before joining any partnership, **ensure** you have the **same work ethos** as your partners

time, then you don't want to find that you have joined a workaholic partnership whose principal interest is maximizing profits.

Once you have ensured that you and your potential GP partners are like-minded and get on together, you need to take a close look at the practice accounts to be sure that the practice is financially sound and will support the level of income that has been indicated. You also need to be clear that you understand how much money you will be required to introduce into the business and what this is for. If you are at all concerned about being able to interpret a set of accounts sufficiently well to enable you to decide whether or not to join a partnership, it is advisable to seek a little professional guidance from a specialist medical accountant who, in a short meeting, will be able to talk you through the accounts, comment on the profitability of the practice and point out any pitfalls. This all applies just as much whether you are joining your first partnership or making a subsequent change.

Understanding a set of accounts

A set of accounts is effectively divided into two main sections:
- the income and expenditure account, which shows how the practice's profit in the year has been generated and the allocation of profit between partners
- the balance sheet, which shows the partners' funds invested in the practice and how those funds have been used.

There should be detailed notes to both parts of the accounts giving you all the information you need in order to understand the business.

The income and expenditure account

The income and expenditure account should categorize income and expenses, and give you the comparative results for the previous accounting year so that you can judge how well the practice is performing. You need to be able to see the income split into its various sources so that you can appreciate, for example, how reliant a dispensing practice is on dispensing income, or how much non-NHS income the practice generates. It is worth bearing in mind that although the annual net intended NHS income per GP is £56 510 from 1 April 2001, many GPs earn as much as £90 000–100 000 from their NHS and non-NHS income, while some less profitable full-time GPs earn as little as £30 000. It is therefore worth studying the accounts to see how profitable the practice is. This critical analysis of your practice accounts each year is important to ensure that you are maximizing the profit of the practice and that it is being managed efficiently.

The balance sheet

It is surprising how many GP partners manage to go through almost to retirement without fully understanding the balance sheet in their accounts. The balance sheet is so called because it is literally made up of two halves that balance (an example is shown in Table 1). One half shows the assets less the liabilities of the practice and the other half shows the partners' funds that are represented by those assets and liabilities.

> Many GP partners manage to almost **reach retirement without understanding** the **balance sheet**

The partners' funds should, ideally, be separated into their constituent parts, being the property capital accounts, practice capital accounts and current accounts (Table 2). In some accounts, this will all be shown together under 'partners' capital' – if this is the case, it is very difficult for partners to know if they have too much or even too little of their money retained in the practice.

Property capital accounts
The property capital accounts represent the partners' investment in the surgery premises. It comprises the value of the property in the accounts less the outstanding partnership loan at the balance sheet date. As a new partner, when you buy into the surgery premises, they will be revalued and you will need to introduce funds for your share of any excess of the value over the partnership loan. This can be done by means of taking out a personal loan for partnership capital; full tax relief is available on the loan interest, but not on the capital repayments.

Capital accounts
The capital accounts represent the money that is needed in the practice to fund the working capital so that the business can function efficiently.

Table 1

An example of a balance sheet

	Current year		Previous year	
	£	£	£	£
Partners' funds and tax provision				
Property capital accounts		216 000		199 000
Capital accounts		35 000		35 000
Current accounts		9 810		8 193
Tax provisions		60 299		55 250
		321 109		297 443
Employment of funds				
Fixed assets		815 000		811 250
Current assets				
Stock of drugs	3 300		3 100	
Debtors	60 025		58 750	
Cash at bank and in hand	71 234		64 278	
	134 559		126 128	
Current liabilities				
Creditors	43 500		38 935	
Due to former partner	950		–	
	44 450		38 935	
Net current assets		90 109		87 193
		905 109		898 443
Long-term loans		584 000		601 000
Net assets		321 109		297 443

Table 2

Partners' capital accounts

	£
Fixed assets excluding premises	15 000
Stock of drugs	3 300
Debtors	60 025
Less creditors	(43 500)
Minimum capital requirement	34 825
Partners' capital (rounded up)	35 000

Current accounts

The current accounts represent the remainder of the partners' funds in the practice and, where capital accounts are shown separately, the current accounts can be fully paid out to the partners when the accounts are approved. The balances on the current accounts are, therefore, the difference between the individual partners' shares of the profit less their monthly drawings and superannuation, and any other payments made on their behalf by the practice.

It is important to remember that the drawings that you will take on a monthly basis from the practice are not a salary, but purely an advance in respect of your share of the profit for the year. As a GP registrar or hospital doctor your salary was your money and was not repayable if there were insufficient profits or funds to pay you. Drawings are quite different; if, when the accounts are drawn up at the end of the year, your drawings exceeded your share of profit, then you would have an overdrawn current account and the balance would be repayable to the practice.

> Monthly **drawings** taken from the practice are an **advance** on your **share** of the **profit** for the year

Clearly then, it is important that the drawings are calculated on a prudent basis on an anticipated partnership profit level that is definitely achievable.

Tax provisions

Where a partnership provides for tax within the partnership, the tax liability is transferred from the current account to the partner's tax provision account to set aside the amount due to the Inland Revenue. This then means that you don't need to worry about providing for tax personally as the practice accountant has calculated the tax due and provided for it within the partnership.

Some practices do not provide for tax within the partnership, but prefer to provide on a personal basis; in this arrangement, you need to take care that you put sufficient money aside to pay your tax. Again you will need advice from your accountant as to how much you should provide and when it will be payable to the Inland Revenue. This is particularly important in the early years as you enter the tax system as a self-employed person.

Understanding your capital account

When you are looking to join a partnership, it is important to ask how much practice capital you will be expected to introduce and also to agree the timescale for the introduction of capital. This should be clearly set out in the partnership agreement and you should ask to see this document before agreeing to join the practice.

The capital should be based on the working capital requirement of the practice, which is the money that any business needs in order to run efficiently, and pay the staff and other bills.

Taking the example of the balance sheet in Table 1, the capital accounts total £35 000. This provides the funds to finance the fixed assets (excluding the surgery premises), which are the:

- computers
- medical equipment
- furniture and fittings
- stock of drugs that have had to be bought by the doctors but which are only reimbursed when used
- debtors, where the debt is the money due to the practice for work done (as it has yet to be received, it is not giving the practice cash that can be spent).

From this figure should be subtracted the sum owed to creditors (i.e. the people owed money by the practice but who have not yet been paid).

The balance sheet only provides a snapshot of the partnership's finances on the balance sheet date; the next day some cash will have been received from debtors and some creditors may have been paid so there is constant movement between items. However, it gives a good indication of how much capital is needed. If there is more capital in the practice than is necessary then there will be more cash in the bank than is needed; conversely, if there is too little partners' capital in the practice then the practice will be overdrawn at the bank.

The capital should be provided by the partners in accordance with their profit-sharing ratios, so that it is evenly provided by all partners and all the partners are involved in financing the practice. This is important as otherwise the partners who have not funded the partnership may find that they are not involved in practice decision-taking.

Profit sharing in practice

When a new partner joins a partnership, it is very common to have a 6-month mutual-assessment period during which time he or she will often be on a guaranteed fixed share. This is not the same as being a salaried partner who is taxable under PAYE as an employee of the practice. A fixed-share partner is a full partner in the practice, accepted as a GP principal by the health authority and taxable as a self-employed individual. At the end of that time, the new partner will switch to being on a profit-sharing ratio, and that share will gradually increase over the next couple of years

> **Capital** provided by the **partners** should be in accordance with their **profit**-sharing **ratios**

until they are on parity with other partners (i.e. equal profit sharing). Most partners attain parity within 2–3 years and at no time should the profit share be less than one-third of the partner on the highest share. For a part-time partner, this is adjusted pro rata so that a half-time partner must not be on less than one-sixth of the share of a full-time partner.

In many practices, certain sources of income are treated as a prior share before the balance of profits is shared in profit-sharing ratios.

Typical prior shares are net surgery income, which is shared between the property-owning partners in the ratios in which they own the property, seniority allowance and postgraduate education allowance (PGEA). You can also come across prior charges that are certain expenses charged to individual partners rather than being shared. Examples of these are locum costs where a partner has had additional leave, or deputizing costs if not all of the GPs use the deputizing service.

Sickness insurance

As a self-employed person, there is no employer to pay you if you are too ill to work. Most partnership agreements will state that a partner can be absent through sickness for a certain period of time, say 3 months, during which time the partnership will bear the locum cost. After that agreed time, the individual will be responsible for the cost of employing a locum and it is therefore important to take out sickness insurance to provide cover for this. It is generally most cost-effective to take out sickness insurance for up to 12 months and then a permanent health insurance policy to cover any long-term sickness after that time.

GPs have tremendous opportunities for saving for their retirement

Pension arrangements

GPs have tremendous opportunities for saving for their retirement. Although you are self-employed, you can nevertheless contribute 6% of your superannuable income to the NHS superannuation scheme and the NHS also contributes to your pension just as it would if you were an employee. This purchases a guaranteed index-linked pension that is based on your dynamized earnings during your working life as a GP – each year's earnings count towards the pension and are multiplied by an inflation factor to convert them into present-day money. However, in order to achieve the maximum pension, it would be necessary to work as a GP for 40 years; it is therefore advisable to consider topping up the basic pension. This can be done through:

- added years
- free-standing additional voluntary contributions (FSAVCs)
- additional voluntary contributions (AVCs)
- personal pension plans.

Added years

You can agree to buy added years by increasing the 6% contribution to anything up to 15%, depending on how many extra years are needed. This is an ongoing commitment so it cannot be varied each year, but it does present the advantage of enhancing all the benefits available under the superannuation scheme; if you were to die or retire early on grounds of ill health then the added years would be treated as having been fully paid to age 60. The benefits enhanced are:
- index-linked retirement pension and tax-free cash lump sum
- death gratuity payable on death in service
- widow/widower's pension
- children's allowance payable if there are dependent children when the GP dies
- enhanced ill-health retirement provisions.

Although GPs can opt out of the NHS scheme and provide for their pension totally through a personal pension plan, this is not recommended. The NHS scheme has excellent benefits that would be very expensive to provide via a personal scheme. GPs should therefore just look at ways of topping up their NHS pension rather than providing a totally alternative scheme.

FSAVCs

FSAVCs are a more flexible alternative to added years – these can be reviewed each year and there is no commitment to pay a contribution. The 6% contribution can still be made up to 15% of superannuable income, but any unused relief cannot be carried forward to another year and payments must be made by 5 April to qualify for tax relief in the tax year. FSAVCs are paid into a personal pension plan and therefore there is no guaranteed pension or other benefits as under the NHS scheme. FSAVCs are only available to GPs who will not have accrued more than 38.1 years of superannuable service by age 60.

AVCs

AVCs are very similar to FSAVCs, but they are run as an in-house scheme so that arrangement fees can be lower. As with FSAVCs, this scheme only produces extra pension and does not increase the lump sum available on retirement.

Personal pension plans

Many GPs earn non-NHS income as well as their NHS income and this can be used as the basis of personal pension contributions. To see the income available to use for a personal pension contribution, calculate the total relevant earnings for the tax year and then deduct the superannuation contributions made in the year grossed up by 100/6.

If you wish to make substantial personal pension contributions in addition to the superannuation contributions, it is possible to renounce the A9 concession. This is the Inland Revenue concession that enables GPs to obtain tax relief on their superannuation contributions despite being self-employed. By renouncing the concession, you will forego tax relief on the superannuation contributions but can then base your personal pension contributions on your total earned income. This will enable you to receive an NHS pension in addition to a full personal pension. This decision can be reviewed each year so that the concession is only renounced for the particular year in which you wish to make substantial contributions.

As GPs have so many opportunities for pension planning, it is important to seek specialist advice to ensure that you make the right decision for your personal circumstances. There are particular opportunities for pension planning in the run up to retirement as the superannuation lump sum can be invested in a personal pension plan. It is, therefore, particularly worthwhile to seek additional advice at this stage if you wish to enhance your income in retirement.

management issues

Dr Stewart Drage, Secretary of the
Middlesex Local Medical Committees

Never before in the history of primary care has it been so essential for GPs to be on top of NHS management issues. This is because never before has management had such a direct influence on our consultations with patients, the organization of our practices and the position of GPs within the healthcare system.

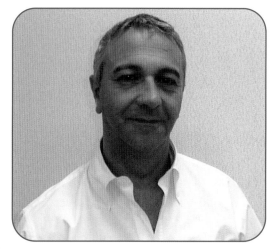

Governments worldwide are grappling with escalating healthcare costs, and the UK is no different. However much money the public is willing to pay, either through taxation or insurance, the costs of providing high-quality standards of care will continue to outpace the funds available, and will do so at an escalating rate as science continues to produce evermore expensive solutions to illnesses.

Add to this the reality that the healthcare budget is determined by Treasury officials and politicians with more than an eye on their parliamentary seats, and it becomes clear why there is so much for them to gain from controlling costs by keeping as much care as they can in the primary sector, while maintaining tight control of the three highest cost pressures:

> Healthcare **costs** are **escalating** worldwide and the **UK** is **no different**

- workforce
- prescribing
- secondary care.

The NHS Plan

To deliver these objectives, the Government has created an NHS Plan for each of the four countries in the UK. It is a management tool of the most challenging proportions. The NHS Plan is being implemented through centrally determined managerial targets and levers at all levels of the service. This includes general practice, where GPs have hitherto been substantially immune from such things, a state of affairs that the Government desires (as did its predecessors) to see radically changed in order, as the jargon goes, to make GPs accountable (to management).

There is very definitely a risk that the solutions posed in the Plan will effectively undermine GPs in their current role. It is for that reason alone that doctors who wish to succeed as GPs need to have a clear understanding of the NHS Plan, and where the managerial risks lie. Of course many of the ideas contained within the Plan may, in the correct circumstances, seem achievable and even laudable. They should, however, be treated with the caution one gives to lighting fireworks. If they go off in the right direction they can be attractive and even breathtaking. If they misfire, their effects can be permanently devastating.

Succeeding as a GP within this framework

To succeed as a GP, you must know how to ensure that your own clinical practice is competently managed, balancing maximum effectiveness with minimal clinical risk. This is the stuff of continuing professional development through life-long learning, personal development plans, the practice, where appropriate, of evidence-based medicine, clinical audit and rational prescribing, and the use of 'tricks of the trade' learned from peers. These should help you to practise high-quality medicine, and will rightly be the fabric of revalidation by the GMC. Under the umbrella of clinical governance they will also, inevitably, be components of the NHS appraisal and performance management processes envisioned in the NHS Plan as part of the system's quality assurance and public guarantee of accountability. As such, it is vital that GPs appreciate how these tools can be misinterpreted, and the potential risks to their livelihood.

Your practice

It is essential to know that the practice as a whole is effectively managed. Employ a good manager, who can implement measures to maintain good patient–staff relations. These should include appraisals, complaints services, good staff-employment practices, and frequent and relevant training programmes. Furthermore, your manager needs to demonstrate effective management of change and organizational development, and should be capable of running an efficient practice that provides a high-quality service while generating income.

Your contract

Make sure that you understand the contract under which you are working. For a salaried GP, this should be a straightforward employment contract. The majority of GPs, however, are independent contractors working either to the current national contract for general medical services (GMS) or to a version of a contract for personal medical services (PMS).

> **Understand** the **contract**
> under which you **work**

The GMS contract comprises a national set of terms of service and a national service specification that is, by and large, based on volume. The statement of fees and allowances are known as the 'red book'. The PMS contract comprises a national core of terms of services and a locally negotiated service specification based on both volume and service delivery. Pay from the GMS contract is determined nationally, while pay from a PMS contract is determined by the local unified budget. NHS management is able to use these contracts as tools; masked as a quality issue, GP contractual change features prominently in the NHS Plan, with the aim of obtaining more efficiency and value for money from you. In this regard, the PMS tool is a far sharper one!

The effect of delayering

NHS structures are being reconfigured (as they tend frequently to be) through the fashionable managerial process of delayering. Hospitals have already experienced this after the 1991 changes and now come under the direct control of NHS management as they are accountable to regional offices of the NHS executive. Under the current NHS Plan, primary care trusts (PCTs) are being created from the rudimentary primary care groups, and for the first time ever GPs will be regarded as working within corporate organizations. These PCTs will be accountable to health authorities which, in turn, are accountable to NHS executive regional offices. Once PCTs are firmly established, the NHS Plan signals reductions in the number and changes in the role of health authorities. Taken to its conclusion, the NHS Plan will make GPs working in primary care organizations directly accountable to NHS executive management through regional offices.

In management terms, the only difference between the PCTs and other trusts will be the continuing independence of GPs as they will remain working as contractors and will, therefore, be one step removed from managerial control. For management this is a major challenge, which is why contractual change also looms large in the NHS Plan. Dressed up as a quality issue, aided and abetted by the relentless exposure of untoward events, from Bristol to Shipman, the policy of using contractual change for GPs is, without doubt, designed to strengthen management's position, neutralizing the threat to the corporativism of the organization – its ability to deliver NHS policy and therefore its funding – posed by GPs' independence. There is a crystal-clear equation between performance of the organization (in terms of achieving the standards set out in the NHS Plan), the funding that the organization receives and therefore the funds available for patient care – particularly prescribing and, crucially, GPs' pay.

In conclusion

Many of the NHS Plan's objectives are worthy; for example, the prioritization of the treatment of critical and chronic disease, and the desire to bring equity across the country in terms of quality of care. Unfortunately, many seem unattainable within the 5–10-year timeframe envisioned. Despite this, NHS management will work to ensure implementation, however unrealistic. The successful GPs will be those who understand the issues identified in this chapter, and take the fullest advantage of the opportunities that arise from them, while appreciating the potential risks.

medicolegal matters

Dr David Pickersgill, GP and Chairman of the
Statutes and Regulations Subcommittee of the General
Practitioners' Committee

The medicolegal aspects of general practice are many and complex and could easily justify a textbook of their own. This chapter focuses on some of the important and topical issues that have a bearing on the day-to-day work of the GP.

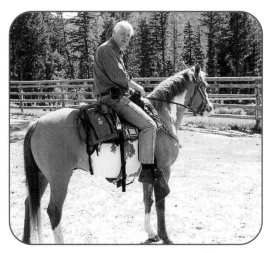

Confidentiality

Personal information can be defined as information about people that doctors learn in their professional capacity, from which individuals can be identified. As a doctor, you have an explicit duty to protect this information – maintaining confidentiality is central to the relationship of trust with your patients.

> Maintaining **confidentiality** is **central to** the relationship of **trust**

Colleagues and employees

You also have a duty to ensure that all those who work with you exercise the same degree of respect for confidentiality. Colleagues/employees should only have access to that part of the information about a patient that is needed in order to perform their specific role in caring for that person. Staff employed by doctors should always have a written contract of employment that contains a clause requiring the employee to understand the need for confidentiality.

Breach

Doctors are professionally responsible to the General Medical Council (GMC) and breaches of confidentiality may constitute grounds for a charge of serious professional misconduct being made.

Legislation and professional recommendations

The issue of confidentiality of health information is covered by:
- the Data Protection Act 1998
- the Access to Health Records Act 1990
- European Human Rights Legislation
- various publications by the GMC, particularly *Confidentiality: Protecting and Providing Information.*

Access to records

The Access to Health Records Act and the implementation of the new Data Protection Act effectively mean that patients have almost unfettered rights of access to their records. The only protection a doctor may have against this is in the provision of the Data Protection Act for a doctor to withhold disclosure of information that may cause harm to the patient, or where disclosure may reveal information about another person and thereby cause a breach of confidentiality to them. You should also take care not to make any entries that you would not wish your patient to see.

> **Patients** have almost unfettered **rights of access** to their **records**

Disclosure to a third party

Disclosure to a third party can occur accidentally when conversations between doctors and staff may be overheard by a third party, or unwittingly in a non-medical setting. Disclosure does, of course, occur frequently with the patient's consent when the doctor corresponds with a third party in order to secure the patient's access to treatment elsewhere in the healthcare system or in supplying information about a patient to bodies such as insurance companies, lawyers and employers. Disclosure to a third party or the patient's representative should only take place with the patient's written consent, or confirmation that the party seeking disclosure has power of attorney over the patient's affairs.

> Disclosure of information without consent should only occur in the most exceptional circumstances

The intentional disclosure of information without the patient's consent should only take place in the most exceptional circumstances. For example, in situations where an individual or the public at large may be placed at risk of death or serious harm. This will include situations such as the disclosure of information to:

- the police in connection with a serious offence, such as murder, rape or child abuse
- the driving licensing authorities when you are aware that a patient is driving while suffering from an illness that makes such action illegal and puts the public at risk.

When faced with a request for information from relatives, a doctor should act with caution, recognizing that although relatives may have a legitimate interest, they do not have a legal right to receive information about a patient without consent. Always ask yourself whether disclosure would be in the patient's best interest; this extends to patients with terminal illnesses.

The duty of confidentiality in relation to medical information extends beyond the death of the patient, and you should not disclose information without the express written consent of the next of kin or the executor of the patient.

Children

Care also needs to be exercised in maintaining the confidentiality of information about children. The Family Law Reform Act 1969 enabled children over 16 to give their own consent to medical treatment. However,

Disclosing information about patients

- Only disclose with the patient's consent
- Ensure that the patient understands
  - to whom disclosure will be made
  - the purpose of disclosure
  - who else may see information after disclosure
- When in doubt, don't disclose, and seek advice from a medical defence organization, the BMA or the General Medical Council

the situation relating to the sharing of information about children under 16 changed as a result of the 'Gillick judgement'. This judgement established a legal precedent, placing an obligation on the doctor to respect a child's wishes if they do not want their parents to know about any proposed treatment, while at the same time obliging the doctor to make reasonable efforts to persuade the child to involve their parents or guardians. As always, your overriding duty must be to do what, in your judgement, is in your patient's best interests.

Confidentiality within the NHS family

Over recent years, the concept of 'the NHS family' has developed and there are those within it who feel that any information about patients can be shared without seeking the patient's consent on each occasion. My recommendations on sharing information are shown in Table 1.

Computer data

Finally, it is worth remembering that with the almost universal use of computers in practices, GPs should be familiar with the provisions of the Data Protection Act 1998. This contains eight principles about the use and storage of data. Further discussion of these principles falls outside the scope of this book, but a code of good practice for GPs, published by the

General Practitioner's Committee of the BMA in September 2000, is available from the BMA.

Consent

"Patients must be given sufficient information in a way that they can understand in order to enable them to exercise their right to make informed decisions about their care" (GMC, 1998).

GPs cannot assume that the registration of a patient with them or provision of care implies that the patient has given the doctor *carte blanche* to impose whatever treatment they feel is appropriate. Having said that, the constraints imposed by the lack of time during GP consultations and the minor nature of many illnesses mean that, in practice, the doctor does not necessarily always specifically obtain the patient's consent to treatment. Nevertheless you have an obligation to present the patient with information about the presumed diagnosis, the implications of that diagnosis and the likely outcome of the illness if no treatment is provided. You should also discuss the need for further investigation when appropriate and the options for treatment, including some mention of any common or serious potential side-effects of the treatment.

> **Patients** must be given sufficient **information** **to make** informed **decisions**

Valid consent

In giving valid consent the following criteria must be satisfied.

- The patient must be competent to give consent.
- The patient must have sufficient information, properly understood, to make a choice.
- Their consent must be given freely.

In helping patients to satisfy these criteria, you should answer their questions honestly and as fully as possible unless the you believe that to do so may cause serious harm to the patient's mental or physical well-being.

In relation to children, the same principles apply as have been outlined in the earlier section on confidentiality.

There are exceptions to obtaining patient consent in relation to patients who are deemed not competent to give it. In the case of adult patients, neither their carers nor the courts have the power to give consent by proxy. In these circumstances, you must act in accordance with what you consider to be in the patient's best interests and must satisfy yourself that such a decision would be supported by a responsible body of medical opinion.

Advance directives

Advance directives may also present some difficulties. Quite frequently, patients will tell their doctor that they do not wish to be treated if they are unfortunate enough to develop a particular illness. If this happens, the patient should be encouraged to put his wishes in writing. If you are contemplating withholding treatment as a consequence of an advance directive, you must be certain that the directive applies specifically to the patient's current condition.

Emergency situations

Not infrequently, GPs have to respond to emergency situations where the patient may not be able to give consent to treatment (for example, a patient who has collapsed). In such a situation, the treatment should be limited to what is immediately necessary to save life or avoid deterioration in the patient's health. Once sufficiently recovered, the patient should be informed about what has been done.

Detailed guidance on this subject is contained in *Seeking Patients Consent: The Ethical Considerations*, published by the GMC in November 1998. This should be compulsory reading.

Medicolegal reports

GPs may be asked to provide factual reports for medicolegal purposes. At the outset, you must be clear as to the use to which your report will be put and the nature of the action in which the patient is involved. If you are implicated in the action, it is imperative that you seek advice from your medical defence organization prior to submitting any report to the patient's solicitor.

Content

A report should begin with a brief summary of your qualifications and career, and the nature of your relationship with the patient. It is helpful if the solicitor's request for a report has set out the specific questions to which a response is required; if this is the case, they should be answered in the same sequence. Comments should be confined to matters of fact; any medical terms should be explained briefly, and opinions expressed only when specifically requested. You should not comment upon, or particularly criticize, the actions of any other doctors who may have been involved in the episode of care under question.

> Providing independent **medicolegal reports** is a **specialist** field

Providing medicolegal reports as an independent expert in general practice is a specialist field, requiring special training and experience.

Medical records

Maintaining good records is critically important (Table 2), which many GPs don't recognize until faced with the need to extract information in response to a complaint or threat of legal action. The nature of GP consultations in the UK and the widespread use of the old Lloyd George records make it difficult, but not impossible, to maintain high-quality records. The introduction of computerized records means that information is held in more than one place and GPs must have access to all relevant information about patients at all times.

Clinical notes serve as an *aide-mémoire* and are also the doctor's most important source of defence should a complaint or legal action arise years later. When a telephone consultation has taken place, questions and responses should be recorded, together with a note of any advice given and an indication of whether the patient or their representative was

Table 2

Medical record-keeping

Records should:
- be legible
- record the date and be made contemporaneously whenever possible
- not use abbreviations that are not in common usage
- have additions and deletions dated and initialled
- indicate that all hospital and laboratory reports have been seen and by whom
- have all correspondence and reports in date order

happy with the advice that was offered. It is wise to record what advice was given to the caller in respect of action that may need to be taken should the patient's condition not improve.

Access

Patients, or their representatives, have legal right of access to both paper and computerized records and you should comply with requests to such access providing they are properly and legally constituted (also see page 118).

Discarding information

It is dangerous practice to discard reports that you consider do not contain any new information or abnormal findings, and it is also dangerous to extract what you consider to be the relevant parts of a consultant's letter and destroy the original.

Complaints

Every GP will be familiar with the NHS complaints procedure, and in particular the requirement to provide an 'in-house' complaints investigation procedure. This must be advertised to patients together with information about how to lodge a complaint and with whom, and how the complaint will be handled. Patients are entitled to ask for their complaint to be investigated by a nominated person in the practice and to receive an explanation within 14 days.

Responding

It is important to acknowledge receipt of the complaint promptly and then cooperate in the detailed investigation, in order to answer as fully as possible all the points that the patient has raised in their letter of complaint. Angry letters should not be fired off by return of post. Refer back to records, speak to any other colleagues or members of staff who may have been involved in the episode of care that has given rise to the complaint, and discuss the proposed response with a colleague or a medical defence organization. Ensure that the response is clear and easily understandable and offer to meet the patient, accompanied if they wish by a friend or advisor, in order to discuss in more detail any of the points in the written response. Also make the patient aware of how they may proceed if they remain dissatisfied with the response.

Many patients register a complaint in order to try to prevent a similar occurrence arising in the future. Be prepared to say in the response what steps have been taken to modify your practice so that such an occurrence will be less likely to occur again. Most importantly, do not be afraid to say sorry – an apology for what has happened does not constitute an admission of fault or blame and it may go a long way to help pacify an angry or dissatisfied patient.

It is worth putting in as much time and effort as possible to satisfy the patient's complaint at this stage as this may well help to prevent the complaint proceeding to formal investigation by the health authority or subsequent legal action.

Clinical negligence

Practising doctors are constantly aware of the increasing threat of legal action arising from an allegation of clinical negligence. There are more than 82 000 incidents of clinical negligence in the NHS each year; a significant number of these arise in general practice, including some of the cases that result in the highest settlements (for example, cases of missed meningitis).

Most cases will be pursued as civil negligence claims, where the claimant must show, on the balance of probability, that he was owed a duty of care by the doctor at the time in question, that the doctor breached that duty of care and that consequently he suffered harm as a result.

The Bolam test

The Bolam test is a standard one that is applied in civil negligence cases; the doctor is not in breach of his legal duty if acting in accordance with a practice 'accepted as proper by a responsible group of medical men skilled in that particular art'. This means that a GP would not be expected to display a greater degree of knowledge, skill and expertise than GPs as a class and he must be able to demonstrate that his actions would be supported by a responsible group of colleagues.

> **Actions** must be able to be **supported** by a **responsible** group of **colleagues**

You must not, therefore, attempt to do things that are beyond your normal level of skill and expertise, and must not delegate duties to colleagues or employees who do not possess the necessary qualifications, skills and experience to perform procedures to a reasonable standard.

Recent years have seen a proliferation of guidelines and protocols for the management of various conditions. Although failure to adhere to this type of guidance is not necessarily negligent, you must be able to justify your actions.

Burden of proof

The courts will determine civil negligence cases on 'the balance of probabilities'; in those cases prosecuted under criminal negligence procedures, the burden of proof is 'beyond reasonable doubt'. The compensation awarded to patients can be very large indeed and, at the time of writing, the largest award made to an individual patient in the UK is £4 500 000.

It goes without saying that if you receive notice that legal action is being contemplated, you should notify your medical defence organization at the earliest possible opportunity and should not respond to any correspondence without taking their advice.

Death certification and cremation regulations

The law requires you, as a doctor, to notify the registrar of births and deaths of the cause of death of any patient whom you have attended during that patient's last illness. This must be done on the form prescribed, stating to the best of your knowledge and belief what the cause is. It is important to realize that this notification is of cause of death and not the fact of death. You are not required to confirm that death has occurred, nor are you required to view the body of the deceased person. Registrars issue death certificates to doctors in the form of a bound book and the book itself contains extensive guidance on completion of the certificates and acceptable terminology. GPs should issue certificates promptly, if only as a matter of convenience for the relatives of the deceased. It is wise practice, whenever possible, to discuss the events surrounding the death with the relatives and give some indication of what cause of death you have entered on the certificate.

> This **notification** is of **cause** of **death** and **not** the **fact** of death

When to report the death

When you are not able to complete the certificate because you do not know the cause of death or when you have not seen the patient within 14 days of their death, you are legally obliged to report the death to the coroner. The coroner, usually acting through one of his officers, will then determine whether a post-mortem examination is necessary, or whether you may complete the death certificate on the basis of your knowledge of the patient's past medical history and taking into account the reported circumstances surrounding the patient's death.

There is much confusion about which deaths need to be reported to the coroner. The fact that a death is sudden or unexpected is not of itself a reason to report the death unless you have not seen the patient within the last 14 days or are unable to satisfy yourself as to cause of death based on your prior knowledge of the patient and the history of events surrounding the death.

Following the revelations surrounding the mass murder of patients by Dr Harold Shipman and the subsequent public inquiry ordered by the Government, it is likely that changes to the regulations regarding the issuing of death certificates will take place in the near future. For the moment, however, if you are in any doubt at all about the cause of death, you are well advised to speak to the coroner's officer before proceeding to issue a certificate.

Referral to the coroner

Registrars are required to refer to the coroner any death where the certificate indicates that there was more than 14 days between the last attendance by the doctor and the death. (In practice, the registrar would normally contact the certifying doctor first and ask whether the case had been notified to or discussed with the coroner. When either of these conditions has been met, the doctor would normally annotate the certificate accordingly.) The registrar must also report to the coroner any deaths where the cause is expressed in vague terms that may imply some doubt, or where they believe the death to have been unnatural, or where the death was due to an industrial disease or industrial poison.

Role of the coroner

The majority of coroners are solicitors working on a part-time basis, though some are full time and some are also qualified in medicine. On being notified of a death that has occurred within the area for which he has jurisdiction, the coroner has to decide whether the circumstances surrounding the death are such that further investigation is warranted. Initially the coroner's officer (usually a police officer) undertakes this investigation, and he will collect such evidence as he feels appropriate and report the circumstances of the case to the coroner. The coroner decides either that a post-mortem examination and inquest are necessary, or that there is sufficient evidence available to issue a death certificate, in which case he will grant permission for the body to be disposed of.

Cremation

Because cremation as a method of disposal of bodies destroys the possibility of any further investigation of the cause of death, additional certificates are required before cremation of the body is permitted. The doctor who has provided the death certificate normally completes the first section of this additional paperwork and a different doctor must complete the second, confirmatory certificate with no professional or family relationship to the first doctor. These two certificates (one piece of paper, in practice) are then scrutinized by the medical officer to the crematorium who confirms that they have been properly completed and provide sufficient information for authority to be given for the cremation to proceed. When a post-mortem examination has been performed, the confirmatory certificate by the second doctor is not necessary. Similarly, when the coroner has been notified and involved, a different certificate (certificate E) will be issued following the post-mortem and GPs will not be involved in providing any further certificates.

> Give due **regard** to the **statement** you are **signing**

If you are called upon to complete the second part of a cremation certificate, you should be fully aware of the obligations placed upon you. You should satisfy yourself that the appearance of the body is consistent with the explanation of the death as given to you by the doctor who has completed the first part of the certificate. You must give due regard to the statement you are signing that you have carefully examined the body and that you are satisfied as to the cause of death.

as others see us

Mr Roy Lilley, Independent Writer and
Broadcaster on Health Issues, and
Former Trust Chair and Health Authority Vice-Chair

An elderly lady, an acquaintance, has been poorly. Nothing terribly serious. Just the routine poorly that you get when your heart has been pumping gallons of blood every day for nearly 90 years. The sort of average indisposition you get when your joints have walked a hundred thousand miles and your back has lifted a million tons in a lifetime of housework and shopping. She's worked all her life, paid her taxes and been a model citizen. She told me she'd been lucky to get an appointment and been able to see a doctor. Lucky? It wasn't her usual doctor. Indeed, she hadn't seen her usual doctor for over a year. "He'd always been too busy". Instead she'd seen a locum, or another partner. On each occasion she had re-told her

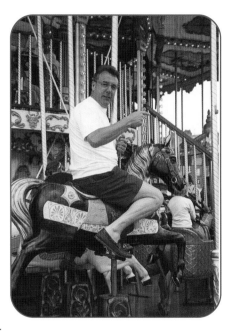

medical history. Lucky? She's been looked after with all the continuity of a rail journey on the East Coast line and with all the insight an interested stranger at a supermarket till could muster. It turns out her GP is the chair of the local primary care group. She would have liked to have seen the familiar face that she relied upon when her husband had gone to sleep for the last time. The man who she thought looked after her children and grandchildren. Now she wasn't sure who did it. A man she had come to see as a friend of the family. Nevertheless, she thought she was lucky.

I don't.

I think she'd been treated in the sort of cavalier way that is the usual preserve of the Post Office. There is no point in clinging to the fond memory of warm beer, vicars on bicycles and a family doctor if one of the family is estranged. If the key member of the family prefers, or is obliged, to be absent, working at the leading edge of medicine with a pile of committee papers, a cup of coffee and ginger biscuit, why dignify the occupation with the words 'family' and 'doctor'.

Another friend is a young blood in the City. Full of energy. Frighteningly dynamic, a terrier, with enough get up and go to make P.-Y. Gerbeau look like a Dome-estic pussy cat. This girl works in the world of domains and dot.coms. She tells me she doesn't bother with her GP. She pays thirty-five quid and pops in to see a doc at the railway station. She tells me she's not been to the local surgery in years. "I get the train at 6.45 am and the surgery isn't open," she said. "I get home around 8 pm and the surgery is closed. Saturdays are just for emergencies (whatever they are) and they're closed on Sundays. So what should I do?" I found it hard to give her advice. Presumably she could go to church on a Sunday and pray for a cure.

> This is a profession **with** few **friends,** some **enemies** and many **undecided**

Having been on the early train, and come home on the late one and found it next to impossible to get a seat, I know she isn't the only one who is probably de-coupling from the NHS. She tells me she can't remember the surgery being open.

So, there you have it. Therein the problem from both ends of the scale.

How did it come to this? How did it all go so badly wrong? Who is to blame? The system? The politicians? Doctors themselves? Who cops for this lot? I guess everyone does. A profession that cannot seem to regulate itself and won't let anyone else do it is a pretty unedifying spectacle. There was a time when politicians busted a gut to protect doctors and stand up for the profession. Even in the teeth of a gale of criticism, ministers would weather the storm and make every effort to calm fears and allay anxiety. Now ministers throw the docs to the dogs. Every week the press-pack feeding frenzy is tossed more fresh medico-malpractice-meat. Ministers can hear the dogs in the yard barking, but they close the door and stay inside. This is a profession with few friends, some enemies and many undecided. Apparently applications to enter medical school are down by 14%.

Where is the noble art of GP-ing, going? I'll tell you. Down-market, down-town and down-the-pan. The technology exists for those with Internet access to self-diagnose most of the common ailments they might want to visit a GP for. The same algorithms that underpin NHS Direct are being sharpened-up for use by non-clinical call-centre staff. Why shouldn't patients have direct access and use them for themselves? The rest is easy. Diagnose, then print off a script and take it to the pharmacist who will double check for appropriateness and contraindications, and the GP is out of the loop.

Women's magazines are, right now, running dial-a-doc services. Readers phone a premium rate number and get access to a GP, 16 hours a day. Web-mobile phone technology will be used for pharmacy and treatment compliance reminders, diet advice and smoking cessation support. Add-in global positioning technology and you'll even know where patients are, which can be useful for the elderly and schizophrenics.

All this tells us there is a medical revolution that will suit the pockets and lifestyle of the middle-classes. Babycare stores will offer health visitor services, charities for the

> This is a **profession** at odds with itself and **overwhelmed** by **change**

elderly will provide subscription services to the growing group in the wealthy grey market. Families will share the cost of a hip-replacement operation for granny, "So she doesn't have to hobble around waiting for the NHS to get its act together." GPs will be left struggling with a population of underclass drug addicts. Battling with self-induced lifestyle-, smoking- and obesity-related diseases that they cannot hope to reduce. Working down-town they risk muggings, assault, break-ins and staff crises. GPs will be suffocating under the avalanche of health management directives pouring out of Whitehall. Crushed by guidelines, treatment protocols, compliance audit and Commission for Health Improvement visits. Strangled in social services' red tape. This is a profession in crisis. I see a profession at odds with itself. A profession overwhelmed by change.

This is a profession that recruits the brightest, from the best schools. Rams them into universities. Force-feeds students on a rich diet, ladled-up by older versions of themselves. They are then released into a world where diagnosing measles for the first time makes them feel like Albert Einstein. By the hundredth time, it is boring and they yearn for something more fulfilling.

But wait. This is also a profession that demands commitment. Obliges attention to detail. Needs a self-belief, extraordinary courage and a level of assurance, to intervene, focus, target, make a decision in a split second and save a life. One that makes being a top-gun pilot look tame. This is a profession that always commands the highest ratings for public trust and honesty. This is a profession where, despite the never-ending stream of bad publicity, still has its waiting rooms full of the hopeful and the bewildered. The architecture of healthcare is changing and many of the participants are ancient monuments.

> There is **no such thing** as 'the profession'. It is the **individuals** that **deliver** the healthcare

What does a young doctor do to point their career in a different direction, to plot a new landscape? Is it possible?

The answer is yes. Yes, not because it is easy, or obvious, but yes because it is vital and no other answer will do. Throwing in the keys to the gate that the profession has guarded so diligently for 50 years is not an option.

In truth, there is no such thing as 'the profession'. It is the individuals that deliver the healthcare, at the bedside, late at night, by the roadside, in a congested surgery. The trick is to bring your expectations to work. The real world you leave behind when you go to work is the world that your patients inhabit all the time.

The NHS is mesmerized by hyperactivity, this initiative, that initiative, one after the other.

Stop ... Think.

Think about creating hell in a restaurant if a wine glass is dirty. Then pause and reflect on the numbers of patients who catch, and die from, hospital- and surgery-acquired infections. Consider for a moment, claiming compensation for a late train. Put that into the context of a patient having to take time off work, to keep an appointment for their healthcare, only to be kept waiting. Remember the last time you returned shoddy goods to a shop and the assistant apologized and replaced the item. Now imagine how a complaint is handled in a busy surgery, by a poorly-trained receptionist.

One person can make a difference. Knowing, acknowledging and admitting a service is poor, unresponsive and stuck in the 1960s is not the same as accepting it. Talking to patients about their expectations is to elevate them to the status of customers. And that is what they are. They, or their family, or all of us, have paid the fees through our taxes and are entitled to be treated as patrons and not patients.

I see a profession at a tipping-point of public opinion. A public hovering with the benefit of the doubt. Doctors wanting it to be all right.

> Be **passionate** about **excellence.** Lead by **example** and **influence** others

Be passionate about excellence, fanatical about customers and their needs, and an enthusiast for transparency and openness. It isn't easy, particularly in a profession marked out for its Masonic attachment to introspection. Talk, incessantly, about modernizing this noble art. Lead by example and influence others.

Above all, remember what it was like to be delighted by a visit to your favourite shop!

The ideal books to help you keep up to date throughout your career

FAST FACTS

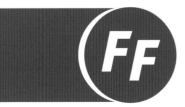

Indispensable
Guides to
Clinical
Practice

Concise, authoritative, accessible, practical information from the *Fast Facts* series of handbooks

A steadily expanding list of titles to give comprehensive coverage of all areas of medicine

Frequent new editions of existing titles to keep pace with the latest developments

Fast Facts titles available at January 2002

Allergic Rhinitis
Anxiety, Panic and Phobias
Asthma
Benign Gynaecological Disease
Benign Prostatic Hyperplasia (*third edition*)
Bladder Cancer
Breast Cancer
Coeliac Disease
Colorectal Cancer
Contraception
Depression
Diabetes Mellitus (*second edition*)
Diseases of the Testis
Disorders of the Hair and Scalp
Dyspepsia
Endometriosis
Epilepsy (*second edition*)
Erectile Dysfunction (*third edition*)
Gynaecological Oncology
Headaches

HIV in Obstetrics and Gynaecology
Hyperlipidaemia
Hypertension (*second edition*)
Inflammatory Bowel Disease
Irritable Bowel Syndrome
Menopause
Minor Surgery
Multiple Sclerosis
Osteoporosis (*third edition*)
Prostate Cancer (*third edition*)
Prostate Specific Antigen (*second edition*)
Respiratory Tract Infections
Schizophrenia
Sexually Transmitted Infections
Soft Tissue Rheumatology
Stress and Strain
Superficial Fungal Infections
Travel Medicine
Urinary Continence (*second edition*)
Urinary Stones

Some forthcoming *Fast Facts* titles

Chronic Obstructive Pulmonary Disease
by William MacNee and Stephen Rennard

Dementia
by Lawrence Whalley and John Breitner

Evidence-Based Medicine
by Jonathan Belsey and Kevin Schulman

Infant Nutrition
by Alan Lucas and Stanley Zlotkin

Parkinson's Disease
by Christopher Clough, Ray Chaudhuri and Kapil Sethi

Psoriasis
by Catherine Smith, Jonathan Barker and Alan Menter

Rheumatoid Arthritis
by John Isaacs and Larry Moreland

Stroke
by Martin Brown and Oscar Benavente

Urinary Tract Infection
by Grannum Sant, Timothy Christmas and Margaret Hannan

£12

For credit card purchases phone Plymbridge distributors on 01752 202301

Published by
Health Press Ltd, Abingdon

www.fastfactsbooks.com

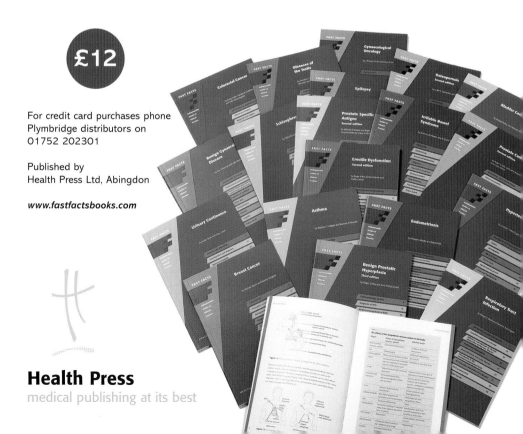

Health Press
medical publishing at its best

www.embarrassingproblems.co.uk
– the website to tell your patients about ...

Based on the BMA-award-winning book *Embarrassing Problems* by Dr Margaret Stearn, this website is the perfect source of authoritative, helpful information for people too embarrassed to discuss health issues.

Winner of the Best Online Consumer Education Initiative in the Global Pharmaceutical Awards, the web site was praised by the judges:

> *"Amazing concept, impressive site,*
> *very good customization, innovative*
> *and dynamic".*

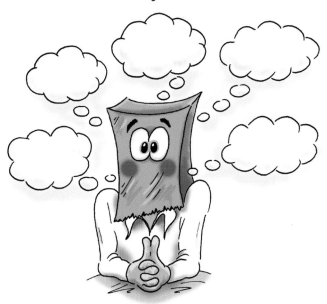

To order copies of the Embarrassing Problems promotional poster for your surgery, simply supply your details and the quantity you require.

Tel: 01235 523233
Email: post@healthpress.co.uk
Fax: 01235 523238